Will Your Children Have Any Doctors?

What You Can Do NOW to Start Fixing Health Care

Karen Ritchie, M.D.

For tomorrow's grandchildren

CONTENTS

Section 4 – Challenges and Questions

"If at first the idea is not absurd,
then there is no hope for it."

Albert Einstein

INTRODUCTION

The last thing Michael remembered was sitting in a jail cell, waiting to be booked. He woke up four days later in the intensive care unit, and learned his heart and breathing had stopped. He had taken an overdose which would have been fatal; however, the police found him in time. They threw him onto the slushy ground, tasered and arrested him. Although he asked to be taken to a hospital, they took him to jail instead.

"Michael" is the pseudonym of an emergency room physician. He survived, and shared his story in a letter to Dr. Pamela Wible.[1] Of his near-fatal suicide attempt, he says, "My decision to end it all was 100% work-related." He likely has post-traumatic stress disorder, from years of dealing with the never-ending trauma and human suffering that passes through an emergency room. The final, triggering event was the death of a young girl with the flu. He had provided appropriate treatment, and his employer expressed support for him, before explaining that he would probably be fired.

If Michael's attempt had been successful, he would have joined the four hundred American physicians each year who suicide. This means we lose the equivalent of two medical school graduating classes every year to suicide alone, in addition to losses from other causes of death. The number of unsuccessful attempts like his is unknown, but is likely many times higher.

"Dr. Jones" is an experienced, caring doctor. His online patient reviews are very positive, averaging almost five stars. He passed his board-certifying exams soon after finishing his training; however, like most doctors, he is required to retake those exams every ten years.

These exams, besides being expensive, are widely considered to be irrelevant. They include many questions that have nothing to do with actual practice realities. Dr. Jones describes them as a game of "medical Trivial Pursuit." The exams have not been shown to improve care, and the vast majority of doctors consider them a waste of time, money, and energy. Dr. Jones, the sole caregiver of a disabled child, did not have the time or money to go to conferences to learn this irrelevant material. He took the exam and failed it. As a result, his hospital terminated his employment. He is now hoping to work as a high school science teacher.[2]

Dr. Stephanie Waggel graduated with her M.D. degree and was in residency training to be a psychiatrist. Despite good evaluations, after she was diagnosed with kidney cancer she was terminated from the program. She was told she was "unprofessional" for going to medical appointments, despite providing advance notice. She offered a note from her own physician, saying that if she had not pursued treatment, the cancer would have been fatal. But she was told by one of her professors, "You need to choose whether you are a doctor or a patient."[3]

These doctors were told they would have to leave the practice of medicine involuntarily. Others are leaving by choice. And though we have a shortage of physicians, it is likely to get much worse. CNN reported that 49 percent of primary care doctors would seriously consider leaving medicine in the next three years if they had an alternative.[4]

A study by the largest physician insurer in the US revealed that nine out of ten doctors would not recommend health care as a profession. The company, describing "vehement, negative reactions" reported that 43 percent said that they were considering retiring within the next five years as a result of changes in health care.[5]

Most Americans realize that the insurance companies and drug companies see us as the enemy, but not everyone understands the demands doctors face. In this book, I describe many of the factors that create an enormous burden on doctors, and why so many of them are leaving the profession. I examine some of the constraints that make practice harder every year, and suck the life out of the doctor-patient relationship.

I make suggestions about what needs to change to allow physicians to simply do our job – that is, taking care of patients. But I also discuss the need to change how we do doctoring. We can't go back to – well, anything, really. The past is gone, and the present state of medical practice is awful. Our only two choices are to keep doing what we're doing, or create something better, more in line with the world we are in now.

I am a physician, but my overall perspective in this book is from the patient's point of view; my ultimate goal is to help people get better. That means doctors need to change some things; we need to change the way we think, and change some of our practices.

Some of the industry's problems can be solved if we stop thinking like a drug company and start thinking like a patient. This means that we need to change what we consider valuable, and change how we look at our information, the literature, and peer review.

I do not see the two perspectives, doctor and patient, as incompatible. If we can bring back humanity and an emphasis on healing to the system, I believe both patients and doctors will benefit.

Although most Americans don't understand the pressures on doctors, nearly everyone knows that our healthcare system is a mess and pleases nobody, except the drug companies. The challenges doctors face are only one of the problems that affect American healthcare – that is, the problems that affect you and me.

Insurance companies charge exorbitant prices, only to deny care they should be covering.

Drug companies lie about their products, distort research information, and spend millions, even billions, of dollars developing "new" drugs that are no better than old drugs.

Doctors rely on our version of science, which we learn about primarily through medical journals. But 50 percent, perhaps as much as 90 percent, of that information is unreliable, or even false. That is not my conclusion, but the conclusion of two editors of the most prestigious medical journals.

For-profit hospitals? I share my experience in Chapter 8.

I have spent many years in various positions in health care, but I have not stayed in one place very long. Looking back, I think I was looking for a healthy place to be, preferably a place that was healthy for me, my colleagues, and the patients. But I rarely found such a place, and if I did, it didn't stay healthy for long. Perhaps such places exist – I hope they do – but I have not found one. My challenge, then, became to stay healthy in a system that seems to get sicker every day.

For the past few years, I have moved from place to place, filling in temporarily where doctors are short, a practice called locum tenens, or "holding the place." Before that, I was the Chief of Psychiatry at M.D. Anderson Cancer Center in Houston, Texas. I am also a bioethicist, with a Masters' degree from Georgetown's Kennedy Institute of Ethics. I was founder and first president of the Midwest Bioethics Center, now the Center for Practical Bioethics.

I worked in private practice, prison, state hospitals, and many outpatient clinics, but for the past few years I have worked with veterans. My goal was to try out an acupressure technique called Emotional Freedom Technique, or EFT, which I found was very helpful for post-traumatic stress disorder (PTSD), among other things.

However, I ran into some problems, not with the technique itself, but with the clinics that claimed to be providing care. The biggest problem was at the facility where I was completely forbidden to use it.

At this hospital, I was working in a clinic for veterans when a veteran I will call Olga came to see me. She had severe post-traumatic stress disorder from her time in the military. She had tried a few medications but had side effects, so she stopped them. Despite her serious illness, she was working full time and was worried about sedation from the medications interfering with her job.

She had difficulty making it to medical appointments because of her work schedule, so psychotherapy was difficult, and her symptoms were so severe that she was unable to take part in the recommended standard therapy protocols for PTSD.

I had been teaching veterans EFT, which is like acupuncture without needles. The veterans were having good success with this technique and asked me to come to their groups to teach others. However, the clinic supervisor, who was not a physician, ordered me to stop using it. This meant that I was ordered not to show Olga the technique that could help her on that day. I considered my options, and decided to obey the order not to teach it to her.

That same evening Olga's symptoms got so bad that she went to the emergency room with a full-blown panic attack. I am convinced that she would not have needed that ER visit if I had shown her how to do EFT.

How did we get to this point, where we are forbidden to use our own medical judgment, where clinical experience is worth nothing, where we take orders from non-physician supervisors more interested in numbers than in people, where we are forced to spend more time on the computer than with patients, and where doctors who can leave the profession are doing so?

What will it take to change this system?

The first question is: who is going to change it? The drug companies aren't going to change it. They are in business to make money, and they are phenomenally successful at doing just that. They have no reason to change.

Congress? Congress does not have an information defi-
cit. Congress has an excess of pharmaceutical lobbyists. Over
1200 drug company lobbyists are registered in Washington,
D.C. alone. That may be why, as I write this, in January 2017,
Congress refused to address the problem of high drug prices.

Dr. Richard Horton, editor of the medical journal *The
Lancet*, reported on a conference of bioscience industry leaders.
They discussed the fact that our current version of science can't
be trusted, that the results are not reliable. The group was clear
that "something must be done." They even agreed that those
present at the conference had the power to do this "something."
But, "The bad news is that nobody is ready to take the first step
to clean up the system."[6]

So, nobody is going to fix this broken system. It's up to us,
you and me. Doctors and patients will have to change it. Health
care reform will have to be crowdsourced.

Reforming the system is an enormous task. It may seem
impossible, but continuing to live with this system is what is
truly impossible. The first obstacle is the enormity of the problem, and our feeling that we are powerless to change it. The
goal of this book is to overcome that obstacle. I describe some
things that you can do now, nine challenges that I see as Step
One. Then I define six issues for Step Two, questions that need to
be answered. For each of these questions, someone, somewhere,
has an answer. If it's you, please share it with us.

So many parts of this industry are dysfunctional, and they
all need to be reviewed. This is not a one-step process, but there
has to be a first step. The insiders are not going to change it, so
we will all have to fix it. That means you, the reader, will have
to start the revolution.

I certainly don't have all the solutions, but I do have a few.
We need to grow a new system. It will take time and needs input
from everyone involved. I hope you will join the effort.

Notes

[1] http://www.idealmedicalcare.org/blog/doctor-revived-suicide-heres-says/

[2] http://www.newsweek.com/abim-american-board-internal-medicine-doctors-revolt-372723

[3] http://www.idealmedicalcare.org/blog/hospital-fires-doctor-for-having-cancer/

[4] http://www.cnn.com/2008/HEALTH/11/17/primary.care.doctors.study/index.html

[5] http://www.thedoctors.com/TDC/PressRoom/PressContent/CON_ID_004671

[6] http://www.thelancet.com/pdfs/journals/lancet/PIIS0140-6736%2815%2960696-1.pdf

SECTION 1

The Problem

"Nearly every month now, another one of
my most brilliant physician colleagues
(from Stanford, Yale, Johns Hopkins, UCLA,
and Harvard) leaves his medical practice."

Melinda Hakim, M.D.[7]

Chapter 1

WILL YOUR CHILDREN HAVE ANY DOCTORS?

After fifteen years of illness, writer Meghan O'Rourke finally had a diagnosis. She had Lyme disease. During those fifteen years, she was in and out of hospitals and doctors' offices. She shared the frustration many patients feel about the health care system, a system that she found insensitive to the needs of patients, gradually eroding the relationship between patient and doctor.

In the November 2014 issue of *The Atlantic*, O'Rourke reviews recent books by physicians, revealing their view of medical practice. She states, "What's going on is more dysfunctional than I imagined in my worst moments. . . few of us have a clear idea of how truly disillusioned many doctors are."

And they are. Doctors are fed up, burned out, and even killing themselves. Many are retiring early, cutting back on work hours, or simply leaving the profession.

O'Rourke quotes Dr. Sandeep Jauhar in *Doctored: The Disillusionment of an American Physician,* who writes that physicians today see themselves as "technicians on an assembly line," or "pawn[s] in a money-making game for hospital administrators." She also quotes Dr. Jack Cochran, executive director of the Permanente Foundation, who visited many clinics and met with "physician after physician" who was "deeply unhappy and often angry."

O'Rourke concludes, "I used to think that change was necessary for the patient's sake. Now I see that it's necessary for
the doctor's sake, too."[8]

Dr. Pamela Wible dated two of her classmates during medical
school. Both killed themselves. In an article titled, "Warning:
Medical school may kill your child," she warns that "Suicide is
an occupational hazard for medical students and physicians."[9]

Doctors kill themselves more than twice as often as non-doc-
tors, and female doctors' suicide rate is twice that of male
doctors.[10]

According to a 2015 article in the *Mayo Clinic Proceedings*,
54% – more than half – of physicians reported burnout, and
the prevalence is increasing. In the authors' definition, "burnout is a syndrome of emotional exhaustion, loss of meaning in
work, feelings of ineffectiveness and a tendency to view people
as objects rather than as human beings."[11]

According to West and colleagues, "Consequences [of
burnout] are negative effects on patient care, professionalism,
physicians' own care and safety (including diverse issues such
as mental health concerns and motor vehicle crashes), and the
viability of health care systems, including reductions in physicians' personal work effort."[12]

This high burnout rate has gotten some attention. Multiple
surveys have found this rate to be consistent, with half or more
of physicians reporting symptoms. Efforts have been made to
address the problem. Various interventions have been attempted
in an effort to change doctors, making them more resilient,
more able to handle the medical world we currently have. But
a focused intervention, presented in the literature as a success,
a pilot program for others to follow, could only reduce the
incidence of burnout from 53 percent to 44 percent. I do not
consider that a success.[13]

The problem is not the physicians. It is not that doctors are
somehow weak or defective or not measuring up. The problem
lies in what we are asking them to do, how we are asking them

to behave, the environment they work in, and the expectations they encounter.

Efforts to teach emotional resilience and emotional intelligence may have merit, but they will not solve the problem. The Mayo clinic researchers recommended changing "contributing factors in the practice environment rather than focusing exclusively on helping physicians care for themselves and training them to be more resilient."[14] In other words, the system itself is causing the trouble, and to focus on "fixing" the doctors is not the answer.

The irony here is that those interventions focus on emotional resilience and emotional intelligence. But the two dominant storylines for physicians are the warrior fighting against death and disease, or the scientist. That is the story of health care, the core of who we are, or at least who we try to be, what we try to do. Both paradigms downplay emotions in the caregiver or forbid them entirely. For the warrior or the logic-based scientist, emotions are merely a nuisance; they get in the way.

Many in the medical profession are proud of being emotionless. This is true of our patients' emotions as well as our own. Doctors are not supposed to have emotional problems, or at least are expected to deal with them on their own, without affecting their performance. Michael, the emergency room doctor with the near-fatal overdose, did not find any support for his PTSD, even though it was caused by his work. Dr. Waggel was distressed that, in a psychiatry department, she was unable to get help with her emotional reaction to having cancer.

At its worst, the industry is cold, soulless, and empty of human qualities. This is not to say that individual doctors are cold, but the industry is making it harder each year to maintain warmth, humanity, and compassion.

This is modeled early in training. Dr. Danielle Ofri, author of *What Doctors Feel: How Emotions Affect the Practice of Medicine* describes the effect the third year of medical school has on students. This is the year they transition from the lecture hall to the bedside, and she describes that they start out altruistic and empathetic, but become jaded and bitter.

"Many of the qualities that students entered medical school with – altruism, empathy, generosity of spirit, love of learning, high ethical standards – are eroded by the end of medical training. . . Much of what they learned about doctor-patient communication, bedside manner, and empathy turns out to be mere lip service when it comes to the actualities of patient care."[15]

Medical students who become disenchanted in their third year may find more of that disillusionment when they finish their training. The model of what medicine is, doesn't match its reality. Taking care of individual patients, doing what that particular patient needs, is not built into the system. Instead, it gets in the way of the process. As Dr. Jauhar described, doctors are turning into assembly line workers. Those who try to be caring and humane are working against the system.

As I think back on my forty-some years in medicine, one image comes to mind. In the original Star Wars movie, our heroes are trapped in the trash compactor. The walls start closing in, making the room smaller and smaller. That is what the practice of medicine over the last four decades feels like to me. In such a room, you start to have trouble breathing, and you know that eventually this will kill you.

The consultation room gets crowded. At one time, it was just me and the patient, and our goal was simply for the patient's health to improve. Now the insurance company is in the room, along with the licensing board and various supervisors and program directors. We are supposed to make them all happy.

Not only are all those folks in the room with us, but their goals are often not the same as our goals. More doctors are becoming corporate employees in order to handle the complicated business and insurance end of medical practice. Increasingly, physicians report to nonphysicians, and those nonphysicians may not understand or care about the things that we care about.

Insurance companies became adversaries long ago; now some administrators and supervisors are becoming adversaries. I have seen doctors write orders that are later reversed by a nonphysician administrator.

A doctor colleague told me a story of sitting at a nurses' station working on a chart. He overheard an administrator talking to the nurse, saying, "You don't *ask* the doctor what he's going to do. You *tell* him what he's going to do." At one hospital where I worked, physicians felt the need to hire an attorney to negotiate a routine employment contract. More than once I have seen a good, well-run clinic, a good place to work, completely destroyed by hiring the wrong clinic supervisor.

I worked with an internist who suggested, mostly in jest, that we change the criteria for admission for medical students. "They don't need to go to college. Just give them a test of their ability to follow directions. Take the ones who are the most obedient. Then give them a phone with all the protocols and they can just follow those."

I am a psychiatrist. Let's say I am seeing a patient who has just suffered a tragic loss. She is crying, and describing to me what has happened. My appointment times are short, as mandated by the organization that employs me, and the next patient is already waiting in the waiting room. I am required to interrupt the patient's story of her child's death so that I can ask her whether she smokes cigarettes. The computerized medical record both demands that I do this, and keeps track of whether I have asked for this information, which is irrelevant to *this* patient on *this* day. If I don't either ask the question and record the answer, or make up a pretend answer, I will hear from my supervisor about it. (The supervisor gets paid more when more of us answer the cigarette question.) The supervisor's followup email, ordering me to call the patient to ask whether she smokes, is titled "Missed Opportunity."

This is not medical care. This is busywork that keeps me from doing good care. It may seem like a small thing, but it's

not a small thing to me, and it's not a small thing to the grieving mother. It interferes with the patient-physician relationship.
And this type of story is repeated with patient after patient, day
after day.

The consumer revolution has changed the practice of medicine. The initial changes were easy to see – sharing information
and requiring patient consent are relatively new. Today's physicians may not believe that not long ago, patients with cancer
were not told of their diagnosis. Research studies must now be
approved by an institutional board convened for that purpose.

But other changes brought by the consumer revolution have
been slower and not as obvious. Access to medical information
has changed the physician-patient dynamic in subtle and not-
so-subtle ways.

Twenty-five years ago, I worked in a cancer hospital. Some
patients would come in with stacks of paper, information about
their disease and potential treatments. They had gotten that
information from a medical library, the only source available
at that time. But not every medical library allowed patients
to use their resources; some did, and some didn't. Now that
information is available to everyone via the internet. And direct-
to-consumer ads for medications provide some information,
although slanted by drug company bias.

Traditional medicine was established with the assumption
that doctors had exclusive access to medical information, and
were the source of information for the patient. But the reality
of information access has changed, and so the doctor-patient
relationship has to change. That change is likely easier for some
doctors, and some patients, than others.

Information access is one change in the doctor-patient relationship. Another is decision-making about medication. Patients
are more likely to demand a certain medication. If a doctor
does not prescribe that medication, the patient will simply go to
another prescriber. I am concerned about the widespread use of
some drugs, such as stimulants like Adderall – I believe we will

eventually look back at this time and conclude that these medications were overprescribed. But patients don't merely request these drugs – they insist on them.

Patients can now leave online reviews of their doctors. While overall this may be a good idea, there are some problems. Patients want many things from their doctors, but many of those things, such as listening, are about treating patients like human beings. These are the very things, as Dr. Ofri has pointed out, that are being squeezed out of medical care. I wanted to listen to the grieving mother, but the clock was ticking and I was supposed to ask her about smoking.

Online reviews are not always objective. An inpatient psychiatrist who treats people who are hospitalized against their will, because they are dangerous to themselves or others, is likely to have biased, often angry and resentful, reviewers. And the goal of making people happy often clashes with the guidelines of our profession and the dictates of our licenses – when people demand opiates, Xanax, or Adderall to fuel an addiction, they are not happy when they are denied.

Notes

7   http://www.huffingtonpost.com/entry/the-alienation-of-americas-best-doctors_us_582899a4e4b0852d9ec218ef?

8   http://www.theatlantic.com/magazine/archive/2014/11/doctors-tell-all-and-its-bad/380785/

9   http://www.kevinmd.com/blog/2016/11/warning-medical-school-may-kill-child.html

10   https://www.ncbi.nlm.nih.gov/pubmed/8833679

11   *More than half of US physicians experiencing professional burnout*; Shanafelt TD, et al. *Mayo Clin Proc.* 2015;doi: 10.1016/j.mayocp.2015.08.023. http://www.healio.com/internal-medicine/practice-management/news/online/%7Bffb4f598-108a-49d1-b569-ead33d6cbbde%7D/more-than-half-of-us-physicians-experiencing-professional-burnout

[12]   Interventions to prevent and reduce physician burnout: a systematic review and meta-analysis, West CP, et al. *Lancet.* 2016; doi:10.1016/S0140-6736(16)31279-X. https://mayoclinic.pure.elsevier.com/en/publications/interventions-to-prevent-and-reduce-physician-burnout-a-systemati

[13]   http://www.thelancet.com/journals/lancet/article/PIIS0140-6736(16)31279-X/fulltext

[14]   Shanafelt, 2016

[15]   http://www.slate.com/articles/health_and_science/medical_examiner/2013/06/medical_school_dark_side_the_third_year_makes_students_less_empathetic.html

Chapter 2

ONCE IS ENOUGH

Physicians have an adversary in their own specialty boards. As *Newsweek* journalist Kurt Eichenwald says, the certifying board for internists "apparently considers itself the enemy of doctors."[16]

Most doctors have a specialty such as surgery, dermatology, or family practice. You have seen the term "board-certified." This means that they passed an exam in their area of expertise. When I was in training, this certification was permanent – you passed the exam once, and were certified for life. The rationale was that either you were capable and proficient or you were not, either/or.

State licensing boards have the task of making sure that doctors *continue* to be competent, that they maintain their skills and continue to be fit to practice. They require a specified number of continuing education hours (called CME, continuing medical education) to keep up on new developments. And if doctors become impaired, those state boards may suspend or revoke their licenses.

When I passed my boards in 1984, this was how it worked. The specialty boards simply verified whether we were capable and knowledgeable at the onset, and the states made sure we continued to be so. Shortly afterwards, this changed. Now, board certification is only good for ten years, requiring doctors to recertify periodically. This requirement is called Maintenance of

Certification, or MOC, and is a major stressor affecting current medical practice.

When recertification was proposed, I thought it was a bad idea; so did many of my colleagues. The change was put through by assuring the doctors of that time that they would continue to be board certified for life, "grandfathered," and recertification would affect only future doctors. We were also promised it would be voluntary.

But MOC has turned into something other than what we were promised. Eichenwald reports that it is so burdensome that it is "harming medicine. A recent report by the National Institutes of Health concluded that, with subspecialty board recertifications becoming more time-consuming, many physician-scientists are refusing to go through the process, choosing instead to drop their hospital privileges and end their work in clinics."[17]

A study published in the *Mayo Clinic Proceedings* polled doctors about their experience with the recertification exams. Physicians in all specialties found the process not relevant and not of value. Eighty-one percent said that MOC is a burden. Only twenty-four percent found it relevant to care of their patients, and only fifteen percent felt it is worth the time and effort (if those who "slightly agree" are excluded, the number goes down to 6.4%.)[18]

What do individual doctors say about the need to periodically retake the board exams? Interviewed at Kidney Week, Lu Huber, MD, a nephrologist in Sioux Falls, S.D., said colleagues and friends told her that "they really vowed to keep their internal medicine certification just because they want to be better nephrologists, but after the MOC [exam], everyone I talked to said, 'I'm not going to do it anymore,' so is it really helping us or doing some harm?"

Stan Nahman, MD, said, "We are not criminals, we want to [get better] at everything we do. I think maintenance of certification (MOC) has just gotten a little out of hand. This idea of [testing to keep] your certification irritates me; you can't take that away from me! I worked like a dog to get certified. Leave me alone!"

Nauman Siddiqi, MD, a nephrologist in Temple Terrace, Florida, said, "To hang everything on a high-stakes exam is what's killing us."[19]

And what of this supposed "voluntary" process? Many hospitals and clinics require current board certification as a condition of employment. Some insurance companies will only pay if the doctor is board certified. And specialty boards are attempting to make board certification a condition of state licensure.

But not in Oklahoma. In April 2016, the Oklahoma House and Senate unanimously passed legislation holding the boards to their claim that MOC is voluntary. In Oklahoma, MOC cannot be used as a "condition of licensure, reimbursement, employment or admitting privileges at a hospital in this state."[20]

This is an active issue, changing rapidly. As of this writing, nineteen state medical societies have passed resolutions opposing compulsory MOC.[21]

The boards claim that recertification is essential to insure quality medical care. But there is no evidence that this is true. And the argument that MOC is important for patient safety has another problem: older doctors like me, whose training was long ago, are grandfathered and do not have to recertify, while younger doctors do. Other prescribers such as nurse practitioners and physician assistants do not have to retest. It is unclear how this policy assures patient safety.

Eichenwald, who is from a family of doctors, believes he knows the motivation for the boards' disconnection from the actual realities of medical practice: money. He has investigated the financial statements of ABIM, the American Board of Internal Medicine, which handles board certification for about one out of every four American doctors. He concludes, "Whooboy, does ABIM have a lot to hide." He explains that the board is in serious financial trouble.

He quotes Charles P. Kroll, a certified public accountant who specializes in health care, who says ABIM's financial statements are "just shocking. . . They are in a financial free fall. I have never seen anything so reckless."

Eichenwald concludes "it is my opinion that the American Board of Internal Medicine (ABIM) has hidden managerial incompetence for years while its officers showered themselves with cash despite their financial ineptitude and the untold damage they have inflicted on the health care system." He believes that ABIM's proposal to increase the frequency of testing to every two or five years is an attempt to fill their financial hole.

One of the complaints about the boards is that so much of what is on the test has nothing to do with what doctors see in their practice. "Videos and study sessions sold to help doctors prepare for re-certification exams often featured instructors saying physicians would never see a particular condition or use a certain diagnostic technique, but they needed to review it because it would be on the test."

As extraneous, irrelevant questions began appearing on the exams, test scores started dropping. The response of the ABIM was that doctors could retake the test. After paying another fee, of course.[22]

Eventually, ABIM made physicians so angry that they have created a competitor, the National Board of Physicians and Surgeons. This board does not require repeat testing, only proof of continuing education, and its fees are much less. Its board is made up of unpaid volunteers.

The main spokesman for this alternative pathway is Dr. Paul Teirstein, who is chief of cardiology at Scripps Clinic. He is quoted as saying, "We don't want to do meaningless work and we don't want to pay fees that are unreasonable and we don't want to line the pockets of administrators."[23]

Dr. Teirstein was invited to debate Dr. Lois Nora, CEO of the American Board of Medical Specialties, the parent organization of the ABIM, at the California Medical Association House of

Delegates in October 2016. Dr. Teirstein's presentation and his Power Point are available here: https://nbpas.org/whats-wrong-with-moc-and-re-certification-by-dr-paul-teirstein/

Dr. Nora declined to publish her video or slides, so it is impossible to tell how her talk was received, but Dr. Teirstein's comments were applauded several times by the delegates. In his presentation, he discusses the fact that many insurers require physicians to have current, renewed board certification. The argument that this insures quality of care is not based on evidence, but according to Dr. Teirstein, is the result of a back-room deal by interlocking governing boards. He concludes that it is about money, not about quality of care at all. It does not benefit patients, but is another burden on doctors. And it is forcing some of them to leave medical practice.

The ABIM certifies one-fourth of American doctors. Other boards seem to have less drama, but are plagued by similar problems. Here is an analysis of the finances of the American Board of Family Practice: http://drwes.blogspot.com/2016/10/the-canary-in-american-board-of-family.html?m=1

This website chronicles efforts to end mandatory MOC for all specialties: http://changeboardrecert.com/

Ending the arduous ten-year exam can be done. The anesthesiology board dropped it in favor of an ongoing continuing education program aimed at learning, not interrogation.[24]

Psychiatrist Dr. Richard Rosin never did get an adequate answer from Dr. Larry Faulkner, president and CEO of the American Board of Psychiatry and Neurology (Dr. Faulkner's annual salary is $843,591). Dr. Rosin wondered why he had to do two MOC's, why diplomates in geriatric psychiatry were required to also maintain their certification in general psychiatry when it was not required of child and adolescent psychiatrists. "Apart from being onerous, this did not seem to be rational, fair, or collaborative." And, he adds, "what if we fail? Has the wand been waved to magically transform us from good to bad doctors?"[25]

Notes

[16]   http://www.newsweek.com/certified-medical-controversy-320495?piano_t=1

[17]   ibid

[18]   http://www.mayoclinicproceedings.org/article/S0025-6196(16)30371-8/abstract?cc=y=

[19]   http://www.medpagetoday.com/MeetingCoverage/ASN/61557?xid=nl_mpt_AACE_confreporter_2016-11-18&eun=g5830087d9r

[20]   https://d4pcfoundation.org/oklahoma-bans-forced-moc-becomes-the-first-right-to-care-state/

[21]   http://rebel.md/state-medical-society-resolutions-against-moc/

[22]   Eichenwald

[23]   http://www.newsweek.com/2015/03/27/ugly-civil-war-american-medicine-312662.html

[24]   http://www.medscape.com/viewarticle/850954

[25]   http://www.mdedge.com/clinicalpsychiatrynews/article/97671/practice-management/ending-moc-nightmare

Chapter 3

ASKING PERMISSION

Dr. Matthew Edlund had tried several medications to treat his patient's depression, and finally found one that worked much better than others. It was a generic – that is, not a brand-name; generic medications are supposed to be less expensive than newer drugs that are still under patent. This medication was not expensive, although it cost a few cents more than the absolute, number one, *least* expensive antidepressant.

He was required to telephone the patient's insurance company to get approval for this generic medication. He had to speak to seven different individuals. Four of them asked him to read off the patient's identifying information: name, social security number, date of birth, address, etc., even though they could see all that information on their own computer screens. This telephone conversation took an hour of Dr. Edlund's time. In the end, the patient gave up on insurance coverage and bought the medication with cash at Walmart.

Another patient did better on a brand-name medication than the generic form, so she wanted to continue it. Dr. Edlund requested approval from her insurer. His secretary spoke to four different people at the insurance company, asking for a preauthorization form that the doctor would fill out by hand. A fax arrived, saying that the next fax would be the form he needed to fill out. But that form never arrived. This happened several times with different patients; a fax requesting a call, which they made, and then a fax saying the next fax would be the requested form. That form never arrived.[26]

Pre-authorization was supposed to be simply a way for insurers to keep their costs down by making sure generic medications were used whenever possible. It has turned into something else.

In a survey of doctors, ninety percent said that the pre-authorization process delays patient access to essential care. That survey showed that the average practice handles thirty-seven prior-authorization requests every week. Seventy-five percent of doctors rated the burden as "high" or "extremely high." The average wait for approval was three business days.

Eighty percent of physicians said that they had to go through the approval process even when a patient has a chronic condition and simply requires continuation of the same medication.

According to the survey, prior authorization is just one of the clerical chores that take about half of doctors' time. This leaves less than 30 percent of the time for seeing patients.[27]

Many doctors just give up rather than spend an hour talking to seven different people. The hassle factor is high. Despite the current push for medical records to be computer-based, prior authorization depends on paper, fax, and telephone calls – slow and inefficient methods that take time away from actual patient care.

One psychiatrist had this conversation with an insurance company representative:

Doctor: I am requesting prior authorization for a medication.
Person on the Other End: What is your specialty?
Doctor: Psychiatry
PotOE: How do you spell psychiatry?

Dr. Edlund concludes, "If you want preauthorization – even for things that cost pennies – we will waste your time. We will tie down both you and your staff so you can't see patients. We will send you on goose chases and down cul-de-sacs you cannot escape. And when you tell patients that we are intractable, we will simply declare it's your fault for "not sending in the form."

We've done our bit. Due process is complete. The lawyers say we're clear."

The insurance companies can certainly review prescriptions to make sure that generic drugs are used when available, as long as there is an appeal for exceptions. Sometimes the prior authorization process will remind the doctor of prescribing problems, such as when two medications have a negative interaction. This is certainly a positive effect of prior authorization.

However, prior authorization comes with a long list of negative consequences. If a medication is not approved that has been working well, the patient must stop taking it. Many medications have withdrawal symptoms that are uncomfortable at least, and sometimes life-threatening. Patients have to wait for refills until approval is granted, an average of three business days and sometimes up to thirty days.

The insurer's list of medications can change, so that a medication was on the approved list last month, and now is not. This is clinically risky at worst, and frustrating at best.

As Dr. Daniel Block points out, "insurance companies are playing a very active role in patient care without carrying any of the responsibility that comes along with being a doctor or other health care provider. . . who is monitoring these insurance companies?"[28]

In a study of patients with Type 2 diabetes, patients whose request for prior authorizations was denied got sicker than those whose request was approved. This resulted in higher medical costs overall, so the denial was more expensive in the end.[29]

As I write this, the AMA is proposing reforms to the process of prior authorization. Let's hope something useful comes from this proposal.[30]

Notes

[26]   https://www.psychologytoday.com/blog/the-power-rest/201511/
       dirty-secrets-health-care-part-ii-preauthorization

27   https://wire.ama-assn.org/practice-management/survey-quan-
     tifies-time-burdens-prior-authorization?utm_source=TWIT-
     TER&utm_medium=Social_AMA&utm_term=807011179&utm_
     content=other&utm_campaign=article_alert

28   http://www.danielblockpsychiatry.com/38/

29   Retrospective Database Analysis of the Impact of Prior
     Authorization for Type 2 Diabetes Medications on Health Care
     Costs in a Medicare Advantage Prescription Drug Plan Population;
     Joette Gdovin Bergeson, Karen Worley, Anthony Louder, Melea
     Ward, John Graham, Jun 2013 Journal of Managed Care Pharmacy
     pp. 374-384c Journal of Managed Care Pharmacy JMCP June
     2013 Vol. 19, No. 5 www.amcp.org

30   https://wire.ama-assn.org/ama-news/21-principles-reform-pri-
     or-authorization-requirements

CHAPTER 4

·························

BUT CAN YOU TYPE?

Three doctors surveyed American physicians to measure professional satisfaction. Initially, their survey did not include questions about the computerized medical chart. But when they interviewed doctors in person, they were so surprised at the intensity of complaints about the electronic health record, as it is called, that they added more questions about it to the survey. They found widespread dissatisfaction and frustration.[31]

The US government has pushed for the adoption of computerized records since 2009, with the intention of improving safety by making records more legible and more available.[32] However, as Dr. David Brailer, the first national coordinator for health information technology, observed, "The current information tools are still difficult to set up. They are hard to use. They fit only parts of what doctors do, and not the rest."[33]

Dr. David Troxel, medical director of a malpractice company, says, "I get more calls from frustrated, angry doctors about their EHRs than any other subject."[34]

When we used a paper chart, only one person could see it at a time. We often had to do patient care without the chart because it couldn't be found, or someone else was using it. In addition, many notes were illegible.

However, with a paper chart, the notes contained what we needed to know. They told us what was important about that individual patient – they would tell the story. To be clear, doctors *already* know what needs to be in a chart note. Our training includes intensive instruction on what we should include, and even what format we should use. We don't need a computer to remind us.

Writing a computerized note can be awkward at best, and nonsensical at worst. Although computer systems vary, for most we can't simply tell the story of the individual patient. We answer questions, many of which are irrelevant. We have to choose between check boxes, and "sobbing mother whose child just died" is not one of those boxes. Real people don't fit into those little squares. As we answer irrelevant questions, we have to stop and think about the answers, often having to figure out the least bad answer. This is a distraction from actual patient care, taking time and attention from what is supposed to be our real job.

If writing a computerized note can be frustrating, reading it may be worse. When we sit down at the terminal we are presented with alerts that can run to several pages. Some of those alerts are crucial information requiring immediate attention. Those are buried in pages of irrelevant, unimportant, or vaguely interesting alerts.

As others have said, "the sheer volume of alerts that range from the "completely irrelevant to life threatening" can "dull the senses, leading to a failure to react to a truly important warning."[35]

And "Irrelevant things are carried forward and more up-to-date information isn't presented."[36]

Reading a note that consists of a long string of check boxes is frustrating and often not helpful. It also does not distinguish between important and irrelevant facts. It leaves me still wanting to know, "what is the story?"

Many doctors are frustrated with having to spend time doing data entry that takes away from time to spend with the patient. Much of what we have to do could be done by clerical staff.

The computerized system does not allow me to document the reality of my visit with the grieving mother. But it does record whether I asked her about smoking. As many clinicians see it, the electronic chart is created for billing and surveillance. It does not serve the purpose of taking care of patients.

The various computer systems don't talk to each other. So doctors must communicate by FAX and phone with other providers or with insurance companies. This incompatibility leads to errors, such as when a pharmacy is on a different system, leading to errors in dispensing medication.[37]

Electronic medical records, as with any computer systems, are liable to crash. They also require downtime for system upgrades, and they are vulnerable to local power outages. Every institution has a contingency plan for such occasions, but those plans can never cover every possible problem.

In the survey of professional satisfaction, electronic health records "were reported as being significantly more expensive than anticipated, creating uncertainties about the sustainability of their use."[38]

EHRs were meant to reduce legal problems but instead, they have created a new, worrisome set of problems. Many systems are not secure – in some, doctors' notes can be altered, either intentionally or unintentionally, by others. The medical record, with its list of check boxes, does not display the limited choices from which the doctor had to choose. It is a poor reflection of the actual clinical care that was provided, but when an issue comes to court, the record is on trial.

The companies that create and sell the EHRs require in their contracts a stipulation that they are not legally liable for any problems that result. This means that the doctor is liable for any problems in documentation that are actually created by the medical record software.

And finally, as health care systems grow, they attempt to get one computerized system that meets the needs of everyone in the system. But as a group of emergency physicians noted, "To think you can take one system and adapt it to those different environments is totally wrong. That's why you see low physician satisfaction and the productivity is going down, all for the sacrifice of having an integrated system."[39]

Notes

[31] http://healthaffairs.org/blog/2014/03/11/physicians-concerns-about-electronic-health-records-implications-and-steps-towards-solutions/

[32] http://www.politico.com/story/2015/05/electronic-record-errors-growing-issue-in-lawsuits-117591

[33] http://www.nytimes.com/2012/10/09/health/the-ups-and-downs-of-electronic-medical-records-the-digital-doctor.html

[34] http://www.politico.com/story/2015/05/electronic-record-errors-growing-issue-in-lawsuits-117591

[35] http://www.modernhealthcare.com/article/20130624/NEWS/306249952/

[36] http://www.politico.com/story/2015/05/electronic-record-errors-growing-issue-in-lawsuits-117591

[37] http://www.nejm.org/doi/full/10.1056/NEJMsb1205420

[38] http://healthaffairs.org/blog/2014/03/11/physicians-concerns-about-electronic-health-records-implications-and-steps-towards-solutions/

[39] http://www.modernhealthcare.com/article/20130624/NEWS/306249952/

CHAPTER 5

A BROKEN SYSTEM

Medical expenses are the most common reason for bankruptcy in the United States. A 2007 Harvard study reported that 62 percent of bankruptcies in the United States were due to medical costs. Of those in this study who filed for bankruptcy due to medical expenses, 77.9 percent had health insurance.

This means that people who were sick enough to require significant medical care, and likely were unable to work, couldn't pay bills and went bankrupt as a result, even though most had health insurance.[40]

If medicine is to "first do no harm," wouldn't this include financial harm?

American health care is the most expensive in the world, by far. According to a PBS report from 2012, the U.S. spends $8,233 per person per year on health care, much more than any other country. The next highest country spends $5,388 per year. The average spending on health care among the other 33 developed countries in the study was $3,268 per person.

U.S. health care costs are now twenty percent of the gross domestic product, GDP. The Netherlands is the next highest, at twelve percent of GDP. The average among the developed countries was 9.5 percent of GDP.[41]

If we are spending the most, much more than other countries, that must mean that we have the best results – that is, we are the healthiest, right?

Well, no. Not even close. According to a *Time Magazine* article from 2014, The United States health care system "has been ranked as the worst among industrialized nations for the fifth time, according to the 2014 Commonwealth Fund survey."[42] The news is all bad. The World Health Report ranked the U.S. health care system 37th in the world. According to an article in the *New England Journal of Medicine*, "In 2006, the United States was number 1 in terms of health care spending per capita but ranked 39th for infant mortality, 43rd for adult female mortality, 42nd for adult male mortality, and 36th for life expectancy . . . [and] the United States is falling farther behind each year."[43]

Our health care expenses are going up but not making us healthier. Clearly, these numbers reflect two different things. One measures health care, what we *do*, and the other, the *results*. Our system is even called a health *care* system, which focuses on what we do rather than the outcome. And what we are doing is not providing the outcome we want. When premiums for mandatory health insurance can be more than house payments and yet we're not the healthiest nation in the world, we need to take another look at what we're doing.

We have a system designed around what we do, what services we offer. I suggest that we change that. I don't believe we will ever have an improvement in health until we make a fundamental change. I propose that we create a system that is designed around the result – *health* – instead of the product – health *care*. I suggest we change into a system that asks, "How can people be healthier?" instead of "What can we do to/for them?"

One example of where we fall down, one reason for the disparity between spending and results, is the problem of chronic illness. By definition, chronic illness is something that our current treatment methods don't resolve. These illnesses persist, becoming a major problem. Diabetes, high blood pressure, and arthritis cause significant discomfort and disability, but our current system doesn't have good answers for these and other chronic illnesses.

Our current health care system is modeled after war. We fight a battle against death and disease, and those who fight the hardest are the heroes. We have had great success with this model against infectious diseases, where the bacteria are the invaders and we fight them off with antibiotics. But this model of the battle doesn't fit well with chronic illness.

We can choose to keep doing what we are doing, or we can fundamentally change our approach. We can keep paying more and more for a system that doesn't resolve the problem of chronic illness or we can do something different. It's our choice. I am suggesting a major change to our assumptions and our approach to health care.

Many proposals for health care reform are like changing the oil on the healthcare vehicle. I am suggesting that we decide where we want to go and then design a vehicle that will get us there. This is not a simple process, and cannot be achieved in one step. But I believe the only way to create a new health system that meets the needs of the payers and the patients – you and me – is to involve us in the process.

What do people actually do?

I live near a drugstore which is part of a national chain. When I am in there I sometimes buy peanut butter cups, along with whatever I came in for. I don't buy malted milk balls, even though they are on the candy shelf, because I don't like them. I just don't like the way they taste. However, some people like them, and clearly people buy them, because the store stocks them.

You don't see me protesting that the store shouldn't carry malted milk balls because I don't like them. However, that is exactly what happens with homeopathic products. The drugstore carries homeopathic products. They carry those products because people buy them, and people buy them because they find them effective.

Some folks strongly object to the fact that well-known chain drugstores carry homeopathic products. I assume these people are well-meaning. They aren't claiming that the products are dangerous or harmful – just the opposite. They claim that the products don't do anything, and therefore shouldn't be carried in the stores.

I will deal with the question of scientific evidence at length in chapter 10. For now, my point is simply that people – a lot of people - buy and use homeopathic products. They also go to practitioners who are not allopathic. Allopathic practitioners are those who use pills, surgery, chemotherapy, etc.; treatment that is covered by health insurance. (Or, that is *supposed* to be covered by insurance. More on the insurance issue later.)

In fact, a 1998 study in the *Journal of the American Medical Association* found that between 1990 and 1997 there was a 47.3% increase in total visits to alternative medicine practitioners, from 427 million in 1990 to 629 million in 1997. In 1997 there were more visits to so-called "alternative" practitioners than total visits to all US primary care physicians. I repeat, there were *more* visits to "alternative" practitioners than to primary care physicians.[44] One has to ask, then, which is alternative and which is mainstream.

Since that 1997 study, the numbers are muddier due to the increase in internet use. With webinars, online courses, etc., the concept of "visits" is not the same as it was. In addition, many so-called "alternative" practitioners provide education about problems rather than attempting to fix them, so a "visit" is not a good description of the services they offer.

The guiding principle of healthcare

For the past two or three decades, the following has been the foundational principle of medicine: Medicine is science. Scientific truth is discovered by formal scientific studies. In medicine, these are large double-blind studies, preferably done by more than one group of researchers. Anything that does not have this type of evidence is considered "unproven." The practitioner learns about these studies from medical journals and textbooks, or at medical conferences.

The second principle which guides many doctors is, "I cannot recommend anything which is unproven." "Unproven" means false.

Both of these principles are new – when I went into medicine more than forty years ago, they were not universal. And the changes we have seen in medicine have their roots in these principles. They have consequences that affect all of us; they have created the health care industry we have today, along with many of its problems.

This is why we can't just change the oil and rotate the tires on the health care system. We need to decide what we want and create a vehicle that will get us there. Our basic assumptions are causing the problem. And we're paying for this, you and I. We have a right to say how our money is spent.

So, what do people actually do? Some people buy homeopathic remedies, for example, instead of going to allopathic physicians. Some are uneasy about fighting against their own bodies and prefer to work with them. Others just don't like the idea of putting manufactured chemicals into their bodies. Some would rather focus on prevention than fixing a problem after it occurs.

But of those who *do* go to allopathic physicians, some have tried everything on the "proven" list and still have symptoms. Some have side effects from medications. Others can't afford those ever-increasing copays.

So, for those physicians who say, "I don't understand why anyone would use something that is unproven," the list above is your answer. If we as a profession throw up our hands and refuse to work with these people, saying "That's not my job," then we will lose our monopoly.

The medical profession is at a crossroads. The industry is getting farther and farther from what patients want, and more and more patients are going elsewhere. If we continue down this path, nobody benefits. If we change course and modify our goal to reflect what patients want and need, everyone benefits. Well, maybe not the drug companies. But I'll get to that.

To the health care industry, you are your disease. The industry defines its purpose as matching up every disease with its appropriate treatment. But you are you. You are a person, and your disease is only part of who you are. And most of the time your disease is only a *small* part of who you are.

For the industry, everyone with the same diagnosis is to be treated the same. But patients are not all the same. And similarly, doctors are not all alike. Many want to treat the person, not just the disease, but are finding it hard, if not nearly impossible. This only increases their burnout.

My father had high blood pressure. When he was in his eighties his doctor treated his blood pressure so aggressively that he couldn't stand up for very long. Hypertension had one set of criteria – goals for blood pressure that were appropriate for someone in his twenties, but much too low for a man in his eighties. He suffered from this for a few years before he found a doctor (thank you, Dr. David Westbrock) who changed his regimen, and gave him his life back. Doctors got paid more if they reduced blood pressure to match the one-size-fits-all criteria, regardless of whether it was the best treatment for that patient.

When I was in training in the 1970's, many psychiatrists - probably most - would describe themselves as eclectic. That means that they knew a variety of things that they could do for patients; they had several choices of treatment methods. The psychiatrist's job was to pick the one that helped that patient the most, to design an individualized treatment. Insurance paid us for our time, and we would decide how to best use that time for the good of the patient.

We can no longer individualize treatment. Now we are presented with a cookbook, one size fits all. Ordinarily, the insurance company will not pay unless that rigid protocol is followed. And if we don't follow the rules, our license may be called into question.

Back in the day, we were encouraged to think, to be creative. We were to see the patient as an individual and create a treatment designed for him or her. Now creativity has been replaced with obedience.

The industry assumes that your disease is the only important part of you, assumes that you simply want to have a diagnosis made and treatment provided. But that is not all that people want from doctors, or from the health care industry. Traditionally, doctors have provided, at least: information, skill, reassurance, prediction, and validation, and many other benefits, depending on the needs of that patient on that day.

Dr. Arthur Frank, a medical sociologist, had a heart attack at age thirty-nine and was diagnosed with cancer at forty. He eloquently describes his experience of being a patient in *At the Will of the Body*. He explains, "Most medical staff do not have the time to be caregivers, and many may not have the inclination. They provide treatment, which . . . is not at all the same."[45]

Those caregivers who *want* to treat us like people, and *try* to treat us like people, find roadblocks everywhere, from lack of time, to endless paperwork that takes the place of meeting the needs of individual patients.

Time with patients is collapsing. There seems to be just enough time to ask questions from the checklist and do the minimal required notes on the chart. Many of us, like Dr. Jauhar, feel like assembly line workers, just barely able to do the minimum required, to follow the guidelines or else. We regularly have to choose between the welfare of the patient and the strict guidelines of the profession. I had to choose whether to demonstrate EFT to Olga or obey my supervisor's order.

Dr. Frank relates that "Professionals can and do care, but when they do they are acting a bit unprofessional . . . [O]ne medical resident spent some time just letting me talk . . . Later his supervisor advised him that once symptoms and history have been elicited, further talk with patients is considered unproductive."[46]

Notes

40   Himmelstein, D.U., Thorne, D., Warren, E. et al, *Medical bank-ruptcy in the United States, 2007: results of a national study*. Am J Med. 2009;122:741–746 http://www.pnhp.org/new_bank-ruptcy_study/Bankruptcy-2009.pdf

41   http://www.pbs.org/newshour/rundown/health-costs-how-the-us-compares-with-other-countries/

42   http://time.com/2888403/u-s-health-care-ranked-worst-in-the-de-veloped-world/

43   *Ranking 37th — Measuring the Performance of the U.S. Health Care System*; Murray, C.J.L., Frenk, J, N Engl J Med 2010; 362:98-99. http://www.nejm.org/doi/full/10.1056/NEJMc1001849#t=article

44   *Trends in alternative medicine use in the United States, 1990-1997: results of a follow-up national survey.* Eisenberg DM, Davis RB, Ettner SL, Appel S, Wilkey S, Van Rompay M, Kessler RC. JAMA. 1998 Nov 11;280(18):1569-75. http://jamanetwork.com/journals/jama/fullarticle/188148

45   Frank, Arthur W., *At the Will of the Body: Reflections on Illness*, Houghton Mifflin, New York, 2002, p. 49

46   Frank, 101-2

Drug companies treat us like fools, like dupes.
Insurance companies treat us like enemies.
This is an abusive relationship, but we depend
on them and we don't know how to leave them.

Karen Ritchie, M.D.

Section 2

Obstacles to Change

I started medical school in 1970. At that time, Ohio State University was piloting an innovative program for medical education. Before being confined to that windowless lecture hall, we had a month of introduction. This involved going out into the city, visiting hospitals and doctors' offices, children's clinics, and sober houses. The goal was apparently to show us where all this was leading, why we were going through all the schooling, and to give us a head start on picking a specialty. My only memory of that month was riding around Columbus with a city health inspector, learning more about trash collection than I ever wanted to know.

As it turned out, a career in public health was not in my future, but I remember the title of that monthlong program: "The Romance of Medicine."

Medicine certainly has a long and rich history. It is a source of great drama, as television programmers know well. The medical heroes of our past provided us with discoveries and knowledge that transformed the profession and still serve as its base. As with any parent, we owe the fathers of medicine a great debt that cannot be repaid; however, while we respect and appreciate them, we are not obliged to see the world the way they see it.

Our medical system was created by grey-haired white guys sitting in leather chairs, smoking cigars, drinking port, and reading paper newspapers. Their accomplishments are to be honored and appreciated, but we do not need do things the way they did them. We can appreciate the "Romance of Medicine" without being held hostage to it.

Whether or not the healthcare system worked in the past, the past is gone. It is now our task to decide which parts of it are working and which are not, and to overhaul it; to take what we have and make it into what we want.

The first step is to take an objective look at the illusions, habits, and traditions that are keeping the industry sick. Although they may have made sense at some time in the past, they no longer serve us. I won't go into too much detail about the problems holding us back; I would rather focus on solutions. But I want to point out some of those illusions, habits, and traditions that are in the way of change.

CHAPTER 6

DRUG COMPANIES

CBC news recently reported that seniors in Warren, Michigan can take a free bus trip to Windsor, Ontario to buy prescription medications. Warren, like other Michigan cities such as Westland and Dearborn Heights, provides transportation for residents to buy drugs much more cheaply than they could buy them in the United States. Warren Mayor Mark Steenbergh was quoted as saying, "Nobody should have to choose between whether to pay for food or for drugs. Prescription medications are a necessity, not a luxury."[47]

Similarly, tour companies in Arizona such as Especially 4-U provide transportation to Mexico. Day tours from the Phoenix area for $79 promise "drug stores with incredibly low prices." The tour company owner says that when they arrive in Mexico, "everyone heads straight into pharmacies."[48]

One reason for the disparity in medical costs between countries is the cost of medications. The same prescription drugs often cost much more in the United States than in the rest of the world. This is because "Unlike every other advanced country, the United States permits drug companies to charge patients whatever they choose." Drug companies "all price drugs much higher here than in other markets" because "we don't regulate prices, as does much of the rest of the world."[49] This policy is established by Congress. It is explained in large part by the drug companies' lobbyists, 1274 of whom are registered in Washington DC alone.

September 2015 saw a dramatic demonstration of this policy. Turing Pharmaceuticals bought the rights to a drug for toxoplasmosis, a relatively rare but life-threatening infection. Turing raised the price of the drug from $18 a pill to $750. "In Britain, in contrast, GlaxoSmithKline sells the drug for 66 cents a pill, and in India, it costs even less."[50]

Turing's chief executive, Martin Shkreli, was perhaps the most hated person in America, until he was succeeded by the CEO of another drug company, Mylan. Mylan makes Epi-pen, which is essential for a great number of people, many of them children. Some schools are required to keep epinephrine, the drug in the Epi-pen, in stock in case of severe allergic reaction. And the drug needs to be replaced frequently, as it has an expiration date.[51]

"Since 2009, Mylan has jacked up the price of the lifesaving allergy treatment an incredible 15 times. The list price on a two-pack of EpiPens is $609, up 400% from seven years ago."

Mylan's CEO, Heather Bresch, stated "I am running a business. I am a for-profit business. I am not hiding from that." Rising profits are a big reason why Bresch earned nearly $19 million in total compensation last year. And over the past three years, she made $54 million."[52]

While "the price of an EpiPen two-pack has surged to more than $600 in the U.S., . . . in the U.K. a similar pair of injectors costs the state-funded National Health Service 53 pounds ($69)."[53]

Americans pay more than people in other countries for the same medication. But they are often not prescribed the same medications. They are likely to be given newer, more expensive drugs, even though in many cases older drugs have been proven to be just as effective as the newer ones. Many new medications, still under patent so they are priced higher, are "me-too" drugs which only imitate an existing drug.

Advertising to doctors and to patients increases prescribing of these newer drugs. You have seen the ever-present television and print ads. And those ads work – they motivate patients to ask their doctors for the brand-name medication, regardless of whether it is the most effective or the most cost-efficient drug for the problem.

Even when patients are not asking for more expensive drugs, doctors often prescribe them when older, cheaper drugs are as effective. Advertising to doctors is a big, mostly hidden, budget item for drug companies. That advertising is often described as education. Dr. Marcia Angell reports that drug companies spend money on "make-believe education" which is actually advertising.

Since the medical industry's guiding principle is that truth is what is published in medical journals and textbooks, the validity of those publications is crucial. If their information is not accurate, the foundation of the industry is open to question.

However, according to Dr. Angell, "Much published research is seriously flawed, leading doctors to believe new drugs are generally more effective and safer than they actually are."[54]

In the January 15, 2009 issue of the *New York Review of Books*, Dr. Angell stated further, "It is simply no longer possible to believe much of the clinical research that is published, or to rely on the judgment of trusted physicians or authoritative medical guidelines. I take no pleasure in this conclusion, which I reached slowly and reluctantly over my two decades as an editor of *The New England Journal of Medicine*."[55]

She explains that drug companies "sponsor minimal research, prepare journal articles based on it, and pay academic researchers to put their names on those articles. Medical education and communication companies were hired to prepare the articles and find authors. . . They paid authors $1000 to put their names on the articles."[56]

Dr. Angell is not alone in this conclusion. Dr. Richard Horton is editor of the prestigious British medical Journal *The Lancet*. According to Wikipedia, *The Lancet* is the second most prestigious medical journal, after the *New England Journal of*

Medicine. Dr. Horton published an editorial on April 11, 2015 in which he said "Much of the scientific literature, perhaps half, may simply be untrue. . . scientists too often sculpt data to fit their preferred theory of the world."[57]

To recap, medicine is based on science. Most practitioners will only prescribe treatment that is science-based. They learn about those treatments through the medical literature. But the editors of the two most influential journals have said in public that the research in those journals is greatly flawed, and cannot be trusted.

What is the result of the editors' stunning admissions? Crickets. Since Dr. Angell's book *The Truth About the Drug Companies: How they Deceive Us and What to Do About It,* was published in 2004, the only change that I can see is that we are legally required to financially support the industry.

Again, Dr. Horton's 2015 editorial ends with this sentence: "The bad news is that nobody is ready to take the first step to clean up the system."[58]

The insiders aren't planning to make a change. If we don't change it, we will continue to have more of the same.

Notes

[47]   http://seniorliving.about.com/od/lawpolitics/a/canadadrug-trips.htm

[48]   http://www.banderasnews.com/0504/hb-cheapmeds.htm

[49]   https://www.washingtonpost.com/opinions/why-do-drug-com-panies-charge-so-much-because-they-can/2015/09/25/967d3df4-6266-11e5-b38e-06883aacba64_story.html?utm_term=.0c54605d14f0

[50]   ibid

[51]   http://www.nytimes.com/2013/09/08/opinion/sunday/epipens-for-all.html

[52]   http://money.cnn.com/2016/08/29/investing/epipen-price-rise-his-tory/index.html

53 http://www.bloomberg.com/news/articles/2016-09-29/epipen-s-69-cost-in-britain-shows-other-extreme-of-drug-pricing-itnvgvam

54 Angell, Marcia, Introduction, *The Truth About the Drug Companies: How They Deceive Us and What to Do About It* Aug 24, 2004, Kindle edition, Amazon

55 http://www.nybooks.com/articles/2009/01/15/drug-companies-doctorsa-story-of-corruption/

56 Angell, 2004, Chapter 9

57 http://www.thelancet.com/pdfs/journals/lancet/PIIS0140-6736%2815%2960696-1.pdf

58 ibid

CHAPTER 7

······················

THE UNAFFORDABLE CARE ACT

Health insurance for everyone was a priority for President Obama. Through his efforts, we now have what is called the Affordable Care Act, known as Obamacare. Many Americans have health insurance through their employers; all others are required by law to have it. Those who can't afford health insurance premiums are supposed to get financial support to pay those premiums. But it is not working out as intended.

The ACA's supporters trumpet the fact that (almost) everyone has health insurance. But having health *insurance* is not the same as having health *care*. This is an illusion - we are fooling ourselves.

For many, the need to pay for health insurance premiums and deductibles means they can't afford to get health care. The Commonwealth Fund's report of August 2015 found that "47 percent of adults in marketplace plans viewed their premiums as difficult to afford.[59]

In 2009, NBC reported that in New York City, it cost more to buy health insurance than it did to rent a two-bedroom apartment. And health insurance costs have gone up since 2009.[60]

When employers offer health insurance, they often find their employees don't take the option because they can't afford it. As one restaurant worker said, "It's either buy insurance or put food in the house" . . . In 2014, about 7.5 million taxpayers paid a fine rather than buy health insurance, according to a preliminary report by the Internal Revenue Service. That is significantly more than the three million to six million the government had forecast."[61]

Insurance premiums keep going up. NPR reported on "sticker shock" from premium increases in the double digits.[62] Web MD reported a 25 percent increase in premiums for "benchmark" silver plans.[63]

Deductibles are increasing to the point that many people can't use their insurance, which contributes to the decision by many not to buy it at all. "Nearly one-fourth of U.S. workers enrolled in high-deductible plans their employers offered last year, up from 4 percent just 10 years ago. That's a troubling trend because we know that patients with high-deductible plans are more likely to delay or skip recommended care."[64]

The Guardian reports that millennials often struggle to justify the high cost of health insurance they are unlikely to use.[65]

Victor Lipman has a good summary of the financial bind people can find themselves in: "In the good old days, health insurance was an irritant but not a nightmare. If you had high premiums, you had low deductibles. And if you had high deductibles, you had low premiums. Now we have high premiums and high deductibles." He accuses insurance companies of "charging extortionary rates and offering paltry benefits."[66]

Health insurance companies regularly deny care that they are supposed to provide. They make the appeal process intimidating. Much of the required documentation is irrelevant, apparently demanded as a nuisance so people will drop the appeal. Health insurance can be cancelled for incorrect reasons or for no apparent reason, without explanation. Attempts to contact the companies are often frustrating. If an actual contact person's name and phone number is provided, they may not answer the call or the voicemail.

There is no risk to the insurance company - if they lose the appeal, they simply pay the costs that they would have paid in the first place, without interest. Meanwhile, the damage to the policyholder's credit, and perhaps life, is done.

A Bing search of "health insurance nightmare" returned 12,700,000 results. Here are a few of the stories:

Karen Oberg had been treated for terminal lung cancer for seven months at the University of Michigan Health System, when her insurance company said it would no longer pay for her care there and she would have to go to another hospital. Her son John made repeated calls to Total Health Care, forty-eight calls in one day, but was unable to get an explanation. He posted a petition on Change.org, which was signed by187,376 people, looking to reverse the decision. Total Health Care gave conflicting responses, first denying that they had ordered her to switch hospitals. Eventually they reversed the decision and approved Karen Oberg's continued chemotherapy at the University of Michigan. In John Oberg's view, "my mom is being looked at as nothing more than a dollar sign and a statistic to this insurance company."[67]

Jamal Davis lost a job, a car, and home loans due to medical expenses which he thought would be covered by his insurance company. At age 18, he was supposed to be covered by his father's insurance. But after a hospitalization for kidney failure, he was told that his insurance company would not cover the $12,000 bill. He had a part-time job at a fast-food restaurant which did not include insurance benefits. But the insurance company insisted that he did have other insurance and turned the bill over to collections. In the meantime, Davis applied for a job at a bank and was turned down due to a negative credit report – the first time he became aware that the bill had not been paid. He and his mother called the insurance company several times and got several different explanations. Eventually the insurance company said they would send a check, but that check was never sent. He lost the bank job, an auto loan, and a home loan due to the erroneous credit report. The issue was only resolved three years later when a local television station intervened.[68]

Sam Safi's insurance nightmare started when he simply changed his home address. Kaiser Permanente mistakenly listed him as a new member and his premiums increased fourfold. He got a bill for $2700 with no explanation, and then his membership was cancelled. He can't make payments on the website because his new account is not listed there. "Their system has messed up my enrollment . . . I've been trying to get hold of this person for nearly 2 weeks but he will not return any of my calls."

Safi adds, "It's very obvious now that such a large healthcare company such as Kaiser Permanente does not care about its members as much as it cares about making money and profits. I never liked dealing with insurance company and I'll never do. I just want to get all of this behind me and live my normal life again with my family."[69]

History professor Dr. Molly Worthen had not paid much attention to health insurance until she became pregnant. At her first prenatal appointment she was asked to pay a "global fee" up front. The financial counselor was unable to give an estimate of what the ultimate cost would be, suggesting that she call her insurance company. Dr. Worthen called the insurance company, which was also unable to be specific about the pending costs. She asked about the cost of some routine blood work but was told that that "those fees are confidential."

She was told that she "may be required to spend $20,000 per year in coinsurance and deductibles." She concludes that "The problem is not just that these costs are astronomical. It's that they are essentially secret. This is the evil genius of the American insurance system. No one has any information, and no one is responsible."[70]

Time asked people to share their stories about the cost of health care. Alexandria Brooks responded that "People ask me about my bills. I am grateful that I had insurance; however, it is not preventing my credit and finances from being ruined. Such a large deductible despite HUGE premiums paid and the disputes between the insurance and the providers leaves one very vulnerable, insured or not."[71]

Are these isolated incidents? The non-profit Advocacy for Patients with Chronic Illness helps people file health insurance appeals. The organization has about an 85 percent success rate, "which is why we know that insurance companies are denying way too often because we shouldn't be winning as many as we are."[72]

Notes

[59]   http://www.commonwealthfund.org/publications/issue-briefs/2015/nov/how-high-health-care-burden

[60]   http://www.nbcnewyork.com/news/local/NYC-Health-Insurance-Costs-More-Than-Rent-Report.html

[61]   http://www.nytimes.com/2015/10/20/business/many-low-income-workers-say-no-to-health-insurance.html?_r=0

[62]   http://www.npr.org/sections/health-shots/2016/10/07/497029662/rising-premiums-rankle-people-paying-full-price-for-health-insurance

[63]   http://www.webmd.com/health-insurance/20161025/sharp-rise-in-obamacare-premiums-for-2017

[64]   http://blogs.aafp.org/cfr/leadervoices/entry/unreasonable_drug_prices_force_patients

[65]   https://www.theguardian.com/money/2014/apr/06/millennials-obamacare-insurance-cost-health-invincible

[66]   https://www.psychologytoday.com/blog/mind-the-manager/201512/why-health-insurance-is-now-bigger-nightmare-ever

[67]   http://abcnews.go.com/Health/terminal-cancer-patient-center-health-insurance-nightmare/story?id=22302395

[68]   http://www.azcentral.com/story/money/business/consumer/call%2012%20for%20action/2014/04/22/healthcare-nightmares/8032901/

[69]   https://samsafi.com/2016/02/10/insurance-nightmare/

[70]   http://www.thedailybeast.com/articles/2014/10/11/despite-obamacare-us-health-system-still-a-complete-mess.html

[71]   http://healthland.time.com/2013/02/28/readers-respond-your-hospital-bill-nightmares-via-cnn-ireport/

[72]   http://www.nbcconnecticut.com/news/health/Appealing-Health-Insurance-Denials.html

Chapter 8

FOR-PROFIT MEDICINE

The past few years I have worked mostly with veterans at government-run institutions. But recently, I worked a temporary job for a very short time at a for-profit institution. It was a very short stint because I gave notice after two weeks.

I had been away from for-profit healthcare for some time, so the change in patient care that I observed was dramatic. It is no exaggeration to say it was shocking. I felt like the third-year medical student, finding out that the Romance of Medicine is anything but. I had gone from Marcus Welby to RoboDoc.

The institution does what is required to meet all the various requirements – governmental regulations, accreditation policies, etc. – which are vast and ever-changing, an enormous task. I have to give them credit for meeting all those obligations. But their policy is apparently that meeting the regulations equals adequate patient care. And that is what they provide – adequate care. Most of the time.

There, doctors' notes are valuable – the primary product. *Doctors*, on the other hand, are interchangeable, an inconvenient necessity, like furniture or equipment. If they don't act as expected, they are replaced with a newer model. I observed as administrators made plans involving physicians without consulting any physicians, and then were surprised when problems came up. The medical staff meeting was required by regulations; otherwise, it would have never been held. This meeting was an occasion for doctors to be talked down to and scolded. They were never asked their opinion; they were not to speak unless spoken to.

The facility prefers that doctors' loyalty is to the institution and not to the patient, or even to professional standards. When I talked to an administrator about doing good care, I got a puzzled look, and never did get my point across. We were simply not speaking the same language – we were talking past each other. This institution doesn't speak the language of patients.

There was no attempt at continuity of care – patients would be assigned to different doctors on different days. Getting a note written was the only goal. The coordinator of mental health staff, responsible for scheduling, patient assignments, and other medical issues, did not know the difference between a psychologist and a psychiatrist, saying (I am not making this up) "they're the same thing."

Staff turnover was high. Four doctors quit in one week when I was there. A social worker, newly hired, quit after five days. One day the nurses called in sick and nursing supervisors had to work the floor. That day, a large stack of pizzas appeared in the nurses' break room. I assume that some corporate procedure manual suggests providing free food if staff are unhappy. However, if the unhappy staff aren't actually *there* that day . . . well, you get the picture.

There were many problems with working at this hospital, but when I got a text message at 1:30 in the morning on my personal cell phone, demanding a response to a clerical question (I was not on call), that was the last straw. I gave notice the next day.

It is no mystery to me that half of all doctors are burned out, as the humanity has been squeezed out of the system. I had an interesting conversation with two colleagues at this hospital; we each had concluded separately that working at this institution was an abusive relationship. This is when I started thinking of the entire industry as abusive.

"You get what you settle for."

Thelma and Louise

SECTION 3

. . . .

What Needs to Change?

Congress, with its army of drug company lobbyists, is not likely to fix anything unless their back is against the wall and they have absolutely no other choice.

That means that you and I have two options. If we continue on our current path, more doctors will burn out, retire early, or kill ourselves. More cheap-to-manufacture medicines will have their prices raised sky-high. More people will file for bankruptcy because of medical bills. And more of your appointment time with your doctor will be taken up with computer data entry.

The other option is that we can change healthcare. We – you and me. Nobody else is going to do it, so it is left to us.

The first thing that needs to change is our collective sense of powerlessness. If we all believe that we can't do anything, nothing will happen. But, as Henry Ford said, "Think you can, think you can't; either way, you'll be right."

We get used to believing that there is nothing we can do, when the opposite is true. Powerlessness is simply a habit of thought and can be changed. There is always something, no matter how small, that we can do. The first step, the one between feeling powerless and doing one small thing, is the biggest step. It gets easier after that.

You can change how you think about some things. You can change how you speak about things. You can start doing one simple thing every day, or stop doing another.

I have listed some challenges in Chapter 15. Some will be applicable to you, many won't. Some are simple things that you can do now.

Our future, and that of our children, depends on what we do now.

Chapter 9

GPS

I used to carry around a pile of paper maps. Now, instead, I have two GPS systems, one on my phone and one in the dashboard of my car. Each time I turn on either system, I get a warning that says not to rely on it completely. The message says, in essence, "Be sure to look out the window. Check out the road for yourself and don't rely only on me."

The GPS is only a guide, not a master. It gives you suggestions about the correct road, but it is my own responsibility to make sure there is a road there and that the road is open, because the GPS isn't always right. Many times I have gotten directions from a friend who says, "Don't use GPS – it will give you the wrong directions. Here's how you can actually get here."

For doctors, it is exactly the opposite. We are told clearly and repeatedly that what we observe is of no value, an anecdote, subject to observer bias. It is not "evidence." Evidence is only found in those elaborate, expensive drug company studies. Don't look out the window. Pay no attention to the man behind the curtain.

This is ironic, because the heroes of yesterday's medicine were those with powers of observation. They described a disease and got their names forever attached to that disease. History remembers them – Cushing, Hashimoto, Parkinson, Wernicke.

While yesterday's value was clinical skill and observation, today's value is obedience, doing what we are told. This is true not just in medicine; for today's society in general, "Scientists say . . ." is a thought-stopper. At this phrase, we are supposed to stop thinking for ourselves and simply believe what is said next.

A medical school lecturer told us, "Half of what we tell you is wrong. We just don't know which half." The appropriate response to that fact would be humility. In fact, science is always in transition – scientific truths are always temporary. What is absolute truth today will be proven wrong tomorrow. Science is a useful tool, but it is not God. It has its limits, even when done right.

I understand that medical students are still told that half of medical truths are wrong. But they find out in their third year that our actual response is not *humility* but *arrogance*. What is "evidence-based" is considered absolute truth and there is only disdain for anything that is not.

And how do we know what is evidence-based? From the journals.

Perhaps the editors of the two most prestigious journals are mistaken. Perhaps the research they and others publish is actually valid. In the 1990's, Dr. John Ioannidis set out to prove that it was. "I assumed that everything we physicians did was basically right, but now I was going to help verify it," he says. "All we'd have to do was systematically review the evidence, trust what it told us, and then everything would be perfect."

Instead, he found that "much of what biomedical researchers conclude in published studies . . . is misleading, exaggerated, and often flat-out wrong. He charges that as much as 90 percent of the published medical information that doctors rely on is flawed." And "His work has been widely accepted by the medical community . . . Ioannidis may be one of the most influential scientists alive."[73]

It is time for the medical profession to admit that our source of information is broken and cannot be entirely relied upon. I do not have a good answer to what can replace the current system, but I agree with Dr. Ioannidis: "Doctors need to rely on instinct and judgment to make choices, [b]ut these choices should be as informed as possible by the evidence. And if the evidence isn't good, doctors should know that, too. And so should patients."[74]

When I was in training, I did a rotation in pediatrics at Columbus Children's Hospital. I was assigned to what they called the Dispensary Clinic, a walk-in clinic for children. I would see whoever came in, all day, five days a week. By the end of the month, when I walked in the door of the examination room, I could tell at a glance whether the child was "sick" or not. I can't tell you how I knew, but I knew. It is the same when patients are dying. After a while, when you do something all day, every day, you just know. That is clinical judgment. I am not unique in this ability – we all acquire it. To disparage clinical judgment and not take it into account is to diminish the quality of medical care.

Similarly, we are disparaging of intuition, but intuition on the part of the doctor and the patient is a source of information that can be helpful. Yale cancer surgeon Dr. Bernie Siegel famously listened to his patients' intuition, and even did a form of art therapy with them.

Intuition is not 100 percent, but it is not zero, either. In psychotherapy, I would frequently hear a patient say, "I should have listened to my intuition. I knew that wouldn't work." I never heard anyone regret listening to their intuition.

Was my pediatric sense of whether a child was "sick," a form of intuition or clinical judgment? I don't know, and I'm not sure there is a difference. But as inaccurate as our current evidence base is now, we cannot claim that it is better than experience, observation, and judgment. I know that I was a better doctor after that rotation, and I can't tell you now, decades later, whether or not I read any journal articles that month.

Notes

[73] http://www.theatlantic.com/magazine/archive/2010/11/lies-damned-lies-and-medical-science/308269/

[74] ibid

CHAPTER 10

SCIENCE

Medicine's fundamental principle is that we depend only on science. Science is our window to the world, the only reliable source of information. Evidence is truth. All else is nonsense.

But according to Dr. Ioannidis, as much as ninety percent of today's medical "evidence" may be false. And yet we still view it as the ultimate truth, regarding anything else with disdain.

Dr. David Sackett warns that medicine displays "all three elements of arrogance." Those elements are: it is "*aggressively assertive,*" even, at times, enforced by law. The second element is that it is "*presumptuous,* confident that the interventions it espouses will, on average, do more good than harm" and the third is that it is "*overbearing,* attacking those who question the value of its recommendations."[75]

We have made "the evidence" into a religion – we worship it. But science itself does not justify arrogance. Scientific truths are temporary, the best available explanation for data, but only good until something better comes along.

Science contradicts itself on a regular basis. Yesterday's evidence-based proven treatment is tomorrow's disproven thing of the past. The history of medicine is full of such instances; recent examples are the value of mammograms, dental floss, dietary fat. Eggs are bad for us, eggs are good, eggs are bad. The current opiate crisis has many causes, but one contributing factor is that for many years, we were assured that if people had real pain, they would not become dependent on pain medication. Oops, not true.

The question for the industry is how to move out of our arrogance into a respect for the limitations of science.

The truth of scientific research findings depends on

- What question is asked
- Who pays for the collection of data
- What data is ignored
- Whether the data is distorted

What question is asked

This first point is fundamental to the industry. Current research is based on the question: "Is this thing that can be monetized effective?" This is an expensive question, in money, in time, and in health. When we base the entire industry on this question, we are accepting the *drug company's* perspective. I am proposing that we ask a different question, one from the *patient's* point of view: "What will help people be healthier?"

Who pays for the collection of data

We are making some progress with this issue. We more or less know that study outcomes are affected by who paid for and managed the study. We understand that the payer of the study has a vested interest in the outcome. Journals require authors of their articles to report financial ties to drug companies, but those ties continue. We seem to think that disclosing payments from drug companies is the same is removing the conflict of interest, but it is not the same.

According to Dr. Angell, "Bias is now rampant in drug trials. Bias is built into the study design." Drug companies "load the dice to make sure their drugs [look] good." And if the research results are not in favor of the drug, they prohibit researchers from publishing the data.[76]

She also points out that drug companies can and do create their own private research companies for drug studies, but they prefer to use medical school faculty, who are "thought-leaders" or "key opinion leaders."[77] A study of medical school department chairs found that two thirds received departmental income from drug companies and three fifths received personal income. [78] Dr. Angell estimates that payments from drug companies to physicians run to tens of billions of dollars per year.[79]

What data is ignored

As Dr. Angell reported, the drug companies bury studies which show that their drugs don't work or have serious side effects. That is a major source of misinformation. But there is another set of ignored data which is bigger and potentially more important.

In nearly every research study, some people get better without treatment. Clearly, people can and do heal themselves on a regular basis. In the standard research protocol, the proposed treatment is compared to a sham treatment, a placebo. Some people get better on the treatment and some do not. But some get better only on the placebo.

The Harvard Health Letter explains that "For a long time, the placebo effect was held in low regard. If people responded to a suspect treatment, we said it was 'just the placebo effect.' The suggestion was that they had been fooled in some way, and their response was inauthentic."[80]

"Placebo response has always been high, especially in trials of anti-anxiety and anti-depressant drugs, where it regularly approaches 50%"[81]

The health care industry could make an effort to understand the placebo response: how it works, and what we can do to support it. Instead, we think like a drug company: we ignore it, ridicule it, dismiss it, disparage it. We say, in effect, "We know you can heal yourself, but we're going to ignore that."

"The fact that taking a faux drug can powerfully improve some people's health—the so-called placebo effect—has long been considered an embarrassment to the serious practice of pharmacology. . . response to placebo was considered a psychological trait related to neurosis and gullibility rather than a physiological phenomenon that could be scrutinized in the lab and manipulated for therapeutic benefit."[82]

This placebo blindness is expensive, both in money and in health. The Harvard Health Letter suggests, "Research is showing that the placebo effect often seems to be associated with objective changes in brain chemistry. . . Rather than dismiss it, we should try to understand the placebo effect and harness it when we can."[83]

When we use the term "placebo effect" we are thinking like a drug company. When we think like a patient we say "you healed yourself." When we think like a drug company, placebo responders are "the people who ruin clinical trials." And so drug companies are looking for ways to identify placebo responders ahead of time so they can be excluded from drug trials.[84]

I suggest that instead of thinking like a drug company and ignoring the placebo response, we think like a patient. Instead of assuming that problems can only be healed from outside, let's look – *scientifically* – at ways we can heal ourselves. Instead of discounting the ability of our minds and bodies to heal themselves, I propose that we make the placebo effect a matter of research. Let's understand it, how it works, what can strengthen it, and how we can support it. Challenge #8 in Chapter 15 addresses this suggestion.

Whether the data is distorted

We know that drug companies distort study data to improve their profits. [85] But results are often distorted by the researchers themselves. "it's easy to manipulate results, even unintentionally or unconsciously. . . At every step in the process, there is room to distort results, a way to make a stronger claim or to select what is going to be concluded."[86]

What is the incentive for researchers to do this? Because academic researchers are judged on the number of times their research is published, they must compete for publication to keep their jobs. Their publications count for more in the more respectable journals, where "rejection rates can climb above 90 percent."[87]

Scientists need to make their research stand out in order to be accepted for publication. "In recent years, there has been tremendous pressure on scientists to demonstrate immediate and lucrative results, and enormous scorn when they don't."[88]

"Even when the evidence shows that a particular research idea is wrong, if you have thousands of scientists who have invested their careers in it, they'll continue to publish papers on it."[89]

Journals rely on other scientists – peers – to review papers and decide whether they are worthy of being published. But this practice of peer review assumes that academicians are more interested in truth than in their own biases and reputations. It assumes they are open to new truth, whether or not it agrees with their theories. It assumes they can admit when they were wrong in the past. And, as Dr. Ioannidis has explained, these assumptions are not always valid.

Notes

[75] Cmaj august 20, 2002 vol. 167 no. 4 http://www.cmaj.ca/content/167/4/363.full

[76] Angell, 2004, Chapter 6

[77] Angell, 2009

[78] Eric G. Campbell et al., "Institutional Academic-Industry Relationships," The Journal of the American Medical Association, October 17, 2007. http://jamanetwork.com/journals/jama/fullarticle/209192

[79] Angell, 2009

[80] http://www.health.harvard.edu/mind-and-mood/putting-the-placebo-effect-to-work

[81] http://ahrp.org/pharma-efforts-to-bar-placebo-responders-from-trials-wsj/

[82] http://archive.wired.com/medtech/drugs/magazine/17-09/ff_placebo_effect?currentPage=all

[83] Harvard Health Letter, 2012

[84] AHRP, 2004

[85] Angell, 2004

[86] *The Atlantic*, 2010

[87] ibid

[88] http://www.theglobeandmail.com/opinion/in-montreal-a-wee-opening-in-the-closed-world-of-science-research/article33372907/?utm_content=buffer612d1&utm_medium=social&utm_source=twitter.com&utm_campaign=buffer

[89] *The Atlantic*, 2010

Chapter 11

WHAT IS EVIDENCE?

The healthcare industry considers evidence to be only what is proven by elaborate, formal research. This research is expensive and is generally provided only to treatments that can recover that expense.

If we are to think like a patient instead of a drug company, what would we consider evidence? While some patients follow the research and are focused on the journals' version of evidence, I believe that most simply want to get better, without side effects, and for as little cost as possible.

Certainly, for a treatment with high risk and high toxicity, for instance chemotherapy, we want very good evidence that the treatment works. Money for those elaborate studies is well spent. But what about the benign treatment that I was forbidden to teach Olga, which consists of tapping on acupuncture meridians? This treatment has essentially no side effects. If we're thinking like a drug company, we would insist that it have the billion-dollar treatment before we can recommend it. If we're thinking like a patient, if we have seen it work once or twice, we would offer it to everyone who is interested.

The standard of evidence required for a treatment should be equal to its risk, and to its cost, in all the ways cost can be experienced, and all the factors that make up its downside. We need to develop a sliding scale of evidence required for suggesting or prescribing treatment. Those with high risk should require more evidence, and those with low risk should require less. I am suggesting this in Challenge #7 in Chapter 15.

Which Science?

Medicine is based on science; that much is true. But which science? While anatomy and physiology are key for surgeons, the rest of medicine is mostly based on chemistry. We look at medical problems through the lens of chemistry – what medication can affect the disease?

This is thinking like a drug company, which wants to solve all problems with a chemical that can make them money. We imagine that the only way to correct a problem in the body is to affect its chemistry. But chemistry is not the only science, not the only way to promote healing. Physics is a science also.

We acknowledge electricity in some forms – we value EKG's and EEG's, for instance. But other forms of energy are somehow not worthy of consideration. From the point of view of the patient, this makes no sense.

Homeopathic remedies are not chemically active – that is not in dispute. But that does not necessarily mean they have no activity. The homeopathic rationale is that they are energetically active. Their activity or lack of it can be investigated through physics.

Homeopathic treatments are considered "unproven," which in today's medicine, is understood to mean "worthless." But "unproven" usually means that nobody wants to pay for expensive studies, or that any academic scientist who wants to do those studies would soon be out of a job. "Unproven" is not the same as "proven false," but we operate as if they are the same.

This distinction is the basis for Challenge #6 in Chapter 15.

If health care is to change, we need to be honest about our evidence and its accuracy. If we want to be real scientists, we need to change our perspective.

A scientist follows truth wherever it leads, regardless of the politics involved.

A scientist would not say, "I disagree with your conclusions, so I will not look at the evidence."

A scientist would not say, "I don't know the mechanism, don't know *how* it works, so I will ignore your evidence that it *does* work." After all, we used aspirin for one hundred years without knowing how it worked.

A scientist would not assume that today's truth is final.

A scientist would not equate "unproven" with "false." Unproven is simply unproven, with no evidence, or inadequate evidence, to prove whether it is true or false.

Because thinking like a drug company is central to our current healthcare industry, changing that thinking will be difficult, like doing major surgery. But we can't afford to continue what we are doing. It is time to start thinking like a patient.

The Fringe

If science has all the answers, we can afford to ignore the fringe. But it doesn't.

When we have a problem and are looking for answers, there is a difference between "we can do stuff" and "we can solve the problem." Our current status of treatment for chronic illness is "we can do stuff." When we are satisfied with "we can do stuff," we are thinking like a drug company. When we think like a patient, we conclude "this isn't good enough. Let's look somewhere else for answers."

Our current medical industry hinges on (mostly) drug companies paying for research, and peer reviewed journals. This leather-chair tradition sets the bar very high for new information, and makes it very hard for new truths to take hold. And so the best answers, the new treatments for chronic medical problems, are slow in coming.

When the answers are not coming from the center, we have two choices: we can keep looking in the center or shift our focus to the fringe. Future answers will come from the fringe. But it is only the fringe if nobody is willing to pay for the research that will make it scientific. Here is the formula: pseudoscience plus money equals science. If a treatment modality does not have the elaborate, expensive evidence that some doctors demand, perhaps it is because nobody is willing to pay the enormous cost. Does that mean it doesn't work?

Chapter 12

NUMBERS ARE NOT PEOPLE

I was once asked to see an elderly patient with advanced cancer. The oncologist-in-training asked me to evaluate her for depression. I went to talk to her, and found that she was indeed pulling away from people, not very responsive, not eating. But it was clear to me that she was not depressed, but that her withdrawal was part of the natural dying process. While some people experience sudden death, others have a gradual death, and that is what I saw in her. As I was writing the note on the chart, her doctor saw me and said, "She's depressed, isn't she?" I replied that I didn't think she was depressed, but that she was dying. He asked me, "What is she dying of?" I answered that that was really his area of expertise, not mine, and I didn't know the cause, but that she was indeed dying. His response was, "She can't be dying. There is only a twenty percent chance of dying of that."

I have been puzzled by that strange encounter for many years, wondering, "What was that about?" I now have some thoughts. This is an extreme example, and I have not had a conversation like it with another doctor, before or since. But it didn't come out of nowhere. He was giving a voice to our assumptions, stating what the industry officially believes, what doctors are taught, although it is usually merely implied.

To the healthcare industry, numbers are more real than people. Numbers can be trusted. People can't. The medical literature is the source of truth, and actual people with actual diseases behave the way the literature tells us they do.

We try to fit real patients into our categories, which are based on diseases, and when they don't fit, we try to force them. Most of the time this is not because we *want* to, but because we *have* to. We have to give them a number from the list of disease code numbers. Insurance payers require this, and now our electronic medical records require it also. This is a problem in many ways. In psychiatry, as with other specialties, we may not have a good diagnosis after only one visit.[90] It may take two or three sessions, or even more, before we have a solid diagnosis, but we are still required to guess at each visit. And there are many patients who simply don't fit into our categories. That is because our diagnoses are not Eternal Revealed Truth; they are only our best understanding for now, and will be improved on in the future.

When we think like a drug company, we focus on numbers rather than people. We treat disease rather than patients. We emphasize orthodoxy, following the literature, rather than what the patient tells us. We are more interested in the structure, what we can measure and Xray and see with our eyes. We aim at changing the *body*. But people want treatment for their *experience* – pain, depression, nausea.

When we think like a patient, we treat the person, focusing on whatever is going on at the moment. We listen. We connect. It's time to bring back the ability to individualize care.

Notes

[90] Dr. Allen Frances made this point in his excellent book, *Saving Normal: An Insider's Revolt against Out-of-Control Psychiatric Diagnosis, DSM-5, Big Pharma, and the Medicalization of Ordinary Life,* Harper Collins, New York: 2013, p. 221.

CHAPTER 13

FIXING OR HEALING?

I have a confession to make: I am a recovering fixer. I used to try to fix everything. I thought that was my job. Isn't that what psychiatrists are supposed to do?

But when I was in my forties, I made a promise to myself that I wouldn't give advice to someone who wasn't requesting it. It took a while to change, but over time, I've gotten better at not trying to solve someone else's problem when they're not asking for help.

I changed my approach because I began to understand the downside of fixing. When you fix something for someone else, that implies that the other is powerless, unable to solve the problem. Fixing acts on someone or something with no power of their own.

This is the industry model of healthcare. Doctors are supposed to be mechanics, searching for the broken part and replacing or repairing it. The role for the patient is passive compliance. You are the patient, the consumer, the recipient of care. Your job is to wait "patiently."

And fixing is sometimes necessary, when you can't take care of yourself. You need someone to set the broken bone. You need a surgeon to take out the inflamed appendix. You need antibiotics for the pneumonia. But when the cast is in place, your body heals the fractured bone. After the surgeon sews up the skin, your body creates the scar.

Fixing and healing are not the same. Fixing is what someone else does to you. Healing is what the body does for itself. Fixing is done from outside; healing comes from inside. Outsiders can help but they don't do the actual healing. You do that for yourself.

These days, most fixing depends on technology. But historically, humanity has healed ourselves. Healing is natural – it is how people survived on earth for all this time, without all that technology.

Sometimes we need fixing, sometimes we need teaching, and sometimes we just need information. When a health system takes up twenty percent of our economy, it must provide *all* of those, each when it is needed.

Sometimes people do need to be rescued, but I'm always a little uneasy about the doctor-as-rescuer role. Sometimes it's very clear, as the person is completely unable to do things for themselves. Otherwise, I wonder. I much prefer the teacher role whenever it is appropriate.

Our healthcare system needs to be more than just fixing. Insurance needs to pay for self-healing as well as fixing. I believe it would save us money in the long run. And it is probably the only thing that will make a real difference in our chronic illnesses.

Our doctors' "cookbook" is couched in innocuous-sounding words like "quality of care" and "best practices." But besides the fact that these terms are based on flawed science, they prescribe one treatment for everyone, ignoring individual differences. So the doctor adhering to "best practices" lowered my father's blood pressure enough that he couldn't stand up.

This regimentation is killing us, literally. If it continues, we'll get more of the same.

You have probably noticed the recent publicity about opiate addiction, and the recent increase in opiate overdose deaths. You hear a lot about treatment, with the aim to reduce deaths. This proposed treatment would substitute a legal opiate, buprenorphine, for the illegal substances. This strategy has already been tried, with methadone. A review of history reminds us that opium was supposed to be the cure for alcoholism, heroin the cure for morphine addiction, methadone the cure for heroin addiction. And if those had worked, we wouldn't be still looking for the next best treatment. We get into this spiral because we are treating behavior, not patients. The stated aim is to reduce opiate deaths by reducing the use of illegal opiates. This is treating the *behavior*. It is not treating the *patient*.

Patients want, and need, different things, and the same patient needs different things at different times. The only way to meet that need is to listen to the patient. The doctor-patient relationship was once the center of the healthcare industry. Physicians need to reclaim the ability to individualize care for the patient at the time of the appointment. It is time for doctors to take back our story.

CHAPTER 14

DISDAIN

I believe the biggest unrecognized problem facing American health care today is the lack of respect for the body's ability to heal itself. This omission is expensive, both in money and in health. It also contributes to the belief that when we are ill, we are powerless.

Scorn for self-healing extends to any method which is not accepted by the allopathic industry, extends to anyone who recommends it, and anyone who tries it. It even extends to the body, which is thought to be weak and powerless, and to any practitioner who even looks at the evidence. Step a toe outside the doctor box in the direction of alternative methods, and you risk the scorn of your colleagues, insurance companies will deny your claim, and your license may even be at risk.

The allopathic assumption is that the body is stupid and has to be rescued. And when, thinking like a drug company, our research question is "does this thing that can be monetized work?" then anything that is free is, by definition, worthless.

You may think I am overstating the importance of thinking like a drug company. Perhaps it sounds a bit overdramatic. However, I will share with you one phrase that makes my point: when we try a medication and it doesn't work; that is, the patient doesn't get better, we say that "the patient failed the medication." In other words, it is the patient's fault.

This is a common saying, although it was not used when I trained forty years ago, when the drug companies were not as powerful as they are now. This expression really, *really* bothers me, like fingernails on a blackboard. If this is not an example of thinking like a drug company, nothing is. If this book accomplishes only one thing, to get people to stop using this phrase, it will have at least started a change in our language and perhaps in our thinking.

We rely on our version of science, which is synonymous with the medical literature. But that evidence is distorted by the many factors I outlined previously, so that evidence often does not match up with real patients and their experience. Imagine that you have a question about an electronic device, but you can't find the original manual, so you download a replacement manual. But you find that the downloaded manual was for a different device, a device similar to yours but not exactly the same. You can never get an answer to your question because the manual has instructions for something entirely different. In some ways it is helpful, and in other ways it's not, because it's not meant for your device.

This is our medical and scientific literature. It contains some truth, but many errors. Among other things, it is overly optimistic, downplaying or even hiding negative effects. So medications don't do what we expect them to do: they are less effective and have more side effects. The oncologist did not expect a fatality from his medication, because its risk was downplayed. Often long-term use of a medication is not tested, and problems arise over time that we were not warned about. This contributes to burnout, a hidden source of great frustration.

You don't have to see the whole staircase.
Just take the first step.

Martin Luther King, Jr.

SECTION 4

Challenges and Questions

CHAPTER 15

CHALLENGES

You already know that American health care is a disaster. You already know that insurance companies and drug companies see us as the enemy. You probably *didn't* know how many doctors find they are no longer able to practice quality medicine. This system is a mess, and the insiders, those who seem to have the power, aren't going to fix it. If it is to be fixed, it is up to you and me. Health care reform will have to be crowdsourced.

I am proposing some challenges that can be addressed right now; then I list some questions that need to be answered, so we can take the next step toward growing a new health system - one that will meet the needs of patients.

Some challenges are for doctors, others are for all of us. I use the term "citizens" because we are patients only some of the time, but we are citizens all the time.

Challenge #1 – For doctors and patients/citizens - Refuse to be powerless

Many of us are accustomed to thinking we are powerless, but if all of us keep believing that way, nothing will change. You may believe that there is nothing you can do. But you do have options, and your actions can make a difference.

Patients/citizens –

Remember that without us, there would be no insurance companies, legislators wouldn't get elected, drug companies wouldn't have a market. If we refuse to buy insurance from companies that treat us badly, only respectful insurance companies will remain in business. If we barrage legislators with demands that they regulate drug prices, those prices will go down.

We're paying for this dysfunctional system. The Supreme Court has declared that buying health insurance is a tax. But If health insurance is a tax, we are entitled to a say in how it is spent, just as we have a say in how our local government uses our tax money. Otherwise, it is taxation without representation. Our health insurance premiums and payments go to hospitals, drug companies, and the bureaucracy that is an insurance company. We can insist on having a voice in where that money goes.

Doctors

Doctors need to remember that we are essential and we are in short supply. The practice environment is deteriorating, and that affects both us and our patients. If your institution talks to you about resilience, insisting that you keep doing more with less, blaming you, don't believe it.

The problem is not you; it is the system that makes it harder every year to take care of patients. What if we all demanded that institutions allow for better care? What if we publicly identified the obstacles to quality care and eliminated them?

Challenge #2 – For doctors and patients/citizens – Insist on adequate time with patients

We appreciate doctors, nurses, and social workers who treat people like people. But they find it increasingly difficult. If we are to have a health system for actual humans, we need to make it possible for those professionals to do their jobs.

Doctors

What are the obstacles to good patient care? What takes up time on meaningless tasks that could be better spent with patients? What does the bureaucracy do that simply makes your job harder, without improvement in patient health? What are the factors that increase physician burnout?

Have you considered Direct Primary Care? According to Dr. Ryan Neuhofel, "The DPC physicians I've met nearly always possess a passion that has sadly been beaten out of most of my physician colleagues."[91]

Direct Primary Care (also called medical retainer) is a model which bypasses insurance; instead, patients pay a monthly fee. DPC practices allow much more time for patient appointments, and foster individualized care rather than "cookbook" medicine. The Direct Primary Care Coalition provides education and support.[92] Dr. Pamela Wible is an advocate for DPC and works to inform doctors and patients about their options.[93]

Patients

Consider Direct Primary Care. You may want to look at the Direct Primary Care Coalition's website[92] and Dr. Pamela Wible's information.[93]

Ask your doctors if they have enough time with patients to do good quality care. If not, ask whether citizens can do anything to improve the quality of medical practice. You can talk to hospital administrators and legislators, get media attention, write blogs. Remember, you are ultimately paying the bills.

On page 109 is a form you may want to tear out and take to your doctor to begin this discussion. This form says:

> To my doctor:
>   Do you have enough time to spend with patients?
>   I am aware that some physicians are frustrated with the lack of time they have with patients, and with many other

obstacles to providing quality patient care. Clearly, something needs to be done.

I would like to see this change. I would like to be part of the solution.

What obstacles affect you? Is there anything citizens can do to intervene? What can the general public do to change this?

If you have any suggestions about how patients can help bring back the doctor-patient relationship, I would like to hear them. We can write letters and blogs, make phone calls, and contact local media. We can put pressure on legislators and health care executives. You may have some ideas about other things we can do.

Thank you for considering this matter.

Challenge #3 – For doctors

I worked for a while in a hospital where taking good care of patients was not a priority, and physicians had no voice. I concluded that working there was like being in an abusive relationship. When I discussed this with other staff, they had reached the same conclusion.

Are you in an abusive job? if you are in an environment like the one I described, what is the effect of your job on your health, your life, and your family? If a patient told you that they were in a situation just like yours, what advice would you give? What would you recommend they do about it?

What would happen if an institution's entire medical staff got together and made a list of what they needed to take good care of patients – and themselves? Always remember that they can't operate without us. If doctors refuse to work at such places, those institutions will have to change or go out of business.

Challenge #4 – For doctors. Lifetime specialty board certification

Most doctors describe MOC, periodic renewal of board certification, as anything from an annoyance to a nightmare. MOC is a hot issue, and by the time you read this, perhaps it will be resolved. Board renewal is expensive in time, money, and hassle. This burden is driving some doctors out of the profession, a loss we can't afford.

Insurance companies should not be allowed to mandate ongoing board certification in order for doctors to be reimbursed. This cannot be justified – MOC has not been shown to improve patient care. According to Dr. Paul Teirstein, this insurance requirement appears to be a back-room deal between the two boards.[94] You may want to join the "end the MOC" conversation in your specialty and your state. Updates on current efforts can be found here.[95]

Consider the alternative, the National Board of Physicians and Surgeons.[96]

For Grandfathered Doctors

The change from lifetime certification to MOC happened on our watch. We did not object, but allowed it to happen. Granted, we were lied to – we were told it would be voluntary, and it is not voluntary. Still, I believe we owe something to our younger colleagues. Those of us who are "grandfathered" are board-certified for life. Those who came after us deserve the same. Consider helping to end the MOC requirement.

Are you retired? Do you have time to get involved?

Are you in a position of influence? Can you weigh in on this issue and help make a change?

Challenge #5 – Doctors and other medical personnel – Take back our language from the drug companies

If doctors are to take back our story, we need to take back our words. If the industry is to benefit patients, we need to stop thinking like a drug company and start thinking from the patient's point of view. The words we use reflect our perspective.

Pay attention to daily words and practices. Although it is mostly unconscious on the part of doctors, nurses, and other health care staff, we need to make it conscious. When a drug does not work, *never* say "The patient failed the medication." I don't believe this is a trivial matter – I believe words are a powerful reflection of our thinking, and that words also affect our actions.

I once went to a talk that was billed as an academic lecture about a new medication. The speaker was a physician with university credentials. During the entire lecture, he referred to this new medication, not as "the drug," but "the product." Apparently, the drug company wrote his talk.

Don't be that doctor.

Challenge # 6 – For all medical personnel – Think like a scientist

We need to think like a scientist instead of thinking like a drug company. The healthcare industry uses the term "unproven" as an accusation. It is accompanied by disdain, synonymous with "false." If a treatment does not have elaborate, expensive research behind it, we do not use it. This means that anything that is out of patent, can't be patented, or for whatever reason will not make money for the drug companies, is unlikely to get those studies and will not be offered to the patient.

Doctors can wait forever, if needed, for research to be done. But the patient is hurting now and can't wait. Patients have a right to know about potential therapies that are still being investigated. Olga, the veteran I saw, had a right to know that EFT was available and had helped many of her fellow veterans with PTSD.

If we are thinking like a scientist, there is only "proven true" "proven false" and "undetermined."

Challenge # 7 – All medical personnel – Establish graded standards, depending on risk

If we require elaborate proof such as randomized clinical trials before we recommend a particular therapy, we are thinking like a drug company. It means we only offer treatments that make money – that is, expensive treatments. Inexpensive or free treatments are considered unproven and subject to disdain. This is part of the reason we pay more than other countries for health care, but are not as healthy.

Demanding the same level of evidence for a chemotherapy drug with severe side effects as tapping on your eyebrow doesn't make sense. It would be silly, except that it is expensive and it prevents people like Olga from getting care that would help them. When we think like a patient, we use different standards for different treatments, depending on risk. We require more stringent proof for riskier treatment.

We now require different levels of evidence, in a way that is not scientifically defensible. For something that reinforces the beliefs we already hold, we accept flimsy evidence. But for something that challenges our basic beliefs, we require verification from Dr. William Osler himself, returned from the grave; even then, we might not believe it.

The life of Dr. Ignaz Semmelweis has two important lessons. The first, which we have taken to heart, is that cleanliness is very important in medicine. The second, which we have not learned, is that we are too protective of our basic beliefs, refusing to surrender them even in the face of good evidence. Dr. Semmelweis could not explain *how* handwashing worked to prevent infection, so he was not believed. He was fired. Everyone, even his wife, thought he was insane for believing that cleanliness was important for patient care, and eventually he was committed to an insane asylum.[97]

Clinical observation is evidence. We don't have to know *how* something works in order to observe that it *does* work. Thomas Kuhn famously said that major paradigm shifts have to wait until the older generation dies before a new paradigm takes hold. We don't have that much time.

Challenge # 8 – Patients – Demand research on the placebo effect

Whenever you hear the word "placebo," substitute "you can heal yourself."

I believe that ignoring the body's self-healing capacity is the biggest, most expensive unrecognized problem in our current health care system. I propose that we make the placebo effect a matter of research. Let's understand it, how it works, what can strengthen it, and how we can support it.

I am proposing that every government agency, state and federal, that supports biomedical research allocate 5 percent of those funds to basic and clinical research into the placebo effect, its mechanisms and clinical applications, and energy medicine, including acupuncture.

On page 111 is a form you may want to tear out and take it to your doctor. You can make any changes on the form that you want. It says:

> To my doctor:
> The US pays the most for health care of any country in the world, but we are not the healthiest. I believe we can change that.
> I understand that when self-healing occurs in medical research, it is dismissed as "placebo response" and the data is ignored. I would like more of our tax money to go toward learning how the body heals itself. I support research into self-healing and the placebo response, and ways to assist healing.

I am in favor of allocating five percent of all biomedical research funding to understanding the placebo effect, both basic and clinical science, and energy medicine.

I believe doctors can make this happen through their local medical society and state legislature. Perhaps you would be willing to help that change.

Thank you for considering this request.

Challenge # 9 – Citizens – Health Wiki

I am proposing a health wiki. This would be a database of health interventions, their risks and benefits, and the status of the evidence. It would be transparent, available to anyone. It would be open to all, to collect information on what promotes healing.

It would have three categories of evidence: proven effective, proven ineffective, and pending. It would include healing methodologies from other cultures that we have ignored in our ongoing disdain for non-European cultures. Healing methods used for centuries allowed those cultures to survive, and we may benefit from learning about them. If there is little evidence for a particular healing method, that will be apparent in the database, but people can make up their own minds whether to use it.

Notes

[91] http://www.kevinmd.com/blog/2016/09/direct-primary-care-physicians-trying-rescue-doctors.html?utm_content=buffera80ab&utm_medium=social&utm_source=twitter.com&utm_campaign=buffer

[92] http://www.dpcare.org/about1-ccz5

[93] http://www.idealmedicalcare.org/blog/

[94] https://nbpas.org/whats-wrong-with-moc-and-re-certification-by-dr-paul-teirstein/

[95] http://changeboardrecert.com/

[96] https://nbpas.org/

[97] https://en.wikipedia.org/wiki/Ignaz_Semmelweis

CHAPTER 16

QUESTIONS

I am proposing the above challenges as the first step in reforming health care. The next step is not so obvious. Some things need to change, but it is not clear to me how we can make those changes happen.

The following is a list of questions that you may want to consider. I am calling for a national discussion about these problems. Someone has good answers to each of these questions. If it's you, please share them with us.

Question 1

How do we deal with the fact that our medical literature is not valid – we cannot trust what the journals say? What do we replace this with? How do we create a new source of scientific information with better validity and a shorter lead time from research to dissemination?

Question 2

Drug prices in the United States are much higher than in other countries. Even some generic drugs are ridiculously expensive. This needs to stop. How can we change it?

Question 3

Health insurance companies raised rates because not enough healthy people bought in. That is either because they couldn't afford it, or because they thought it would not benefit them. Many, maybe most, of those young and healthy people bought something that was homeopathic or supplements, or went to a Reiki practitioner or some other "alternative" healing modality.

People will stand in line to buy an IPhone. They have to be forced by law to buy health insurance. What is the difference between those products? What if we made health insurance more like an IPhone, something that more people want to buy?

What we have now is not health insurance. It's sickness insurance. If the industry was truly about health, we would have an easier job selling it. What if we integrated the two systems – the fixing industry and the healing industry? How could we go about that?

Question 4

What do state insurance commissioners actually do? Whatever it is, it is not enough. We need to clean up the insurance industry and make sure that the companies work for us. We are paying for it – health insurance premiums are considered a tax by the Supreme Court, so the taxpayers are entitled to a voice in how that money is spent.

Question 5

How can we use technology to improve health, from the patient's perspective?

We have technology to help deliver care, but most are only a better way to do things we have traditionally done, such as monitoring blood pressure and blood sugar. Surgical technology and other fixing enterprises have made amazing progress. Let's do the same for self-healing.

We also want more things that will make health care more convenient. There is already a gadget to put on your IPhone and look into your baby's ear to check for an infection, then send the image to your doctor, avoiding a trip to the office and a half day off work. We want more of that kind of tech.

How can tech make us healthier? How can it improve the patient's experience with health care?

Question 6

Over the decades, I have seen so many drugs go from prescription to over-the-counter. Why is that? If they were too dangerous for you to buy yourself five years ago, why are they safe now?

We need a new discussion about the need for prescriptions, a discussion from the patient's point of view. When someone is on a stable dose of a medication for blood pressure or depression, they must see their doctor simply to renew a prescription. Is this visit really necessary?

Patients change doses, skip doses, stop medications themselves. And we doctors scold them, or even fire them. But they have a right to do this. After all, they're the ones with the problem, and they know how well the medications are working.

How do we justify protecting people from themselves? How do we justify requiring a doctor's prescription for medications? I am not talking about drugs of abuse, which is a more complicated topic, or antibiotics, which have an important public health aspect. I am talking about medications for diabetes, blood pressure, arthritis. We need a new discussion about requiring prescriptions.

Chapter 17

WHAT'S NEXT?

We spend a great deal of time debating the question of how to pay for health care. But we spend a lot of money on things that don't improve our health, and we ignore others that can improve our health but are free or inexpensive. I believe that we can't answer the question of how to pay for the industry until we decide what we are willing to pay for.

We need to change the *health care* system to a *health* system, and focus on what improves people's well-being. The research question would change from "Is this thing that can be monetized effective?" to "What can improve health?"

Evidence required for any process, device, or chemical should be more stringent for those of greater risk, and less strict for those with less risk. That evidence would be available to everyone on a national database.

Creating a new health system needs to be crowdsourced. We need older people, as they may use health care more, so their experience as a patient is not hypothetical, but real. They can keep us grounded to actual realities.

We need young people who can give us a fresh perspective, ideas we had not considered before. Young people think about technology differently. We need technology, not just to improve the way we do the things we have always done, but to do new things, things we never thought of doing before.

We need historians, so we don't make the same mistakes we made in the past. We need to understand how we got to where we are today, and how other cultures solved their health problems.

We need academics to help us figure out how to redo our system of doing science and publishing the results.

We need older physicians who remember what it was like to practice medicine when we had time with our patients, and could treat them as individuals.

And we need your input.

We need a collective brainstorm and problem-solving project. I can imagine individuals and groups, each picking one issue to focus on; university departments, nursing schools, fourteen-year-old techies. Each could host a forum or working group; publish a blog, brainstorm by videochat, collect opinions and suggestions, hold a contest for the best idea.

My goal for this book is to convince you, the reader, that you can do something to begin fixing this national disaster that is our health care system. Nothing will change unless you and I change it.

For every one of my ideas, someone has a better idea. If it's you, please share it with us.

ACKNOWLEDGEMENTS

I am grateful to my parents, Malcolm and Roberta Ritchie, for their example and their unwavering support. And thanks to Megan, Matt, and Chad for everything. I am truly blessed.

The idea for this book came during a Tom Bird workshop for authors. I benefitted from using Tom's method, and I appreciate the assistance of his staff, especially Sabrina and John.

Dr. Genevieve Yancey and Dr. Kathy Cowan reviewed parts of this book and provided helpful feedback. I appreciate their time and contribution.

I am grateful to my mentors in the medical field for teaching me what medicine can be like, and to the patients who made sure I learned other important lessons! Special thanks to America's doctors, who struggle under a system that makes it ever harder to take care of patients. I am glad you have persevered, but now Let's Fix Health Care!

GLOSSARY

Alerts – When a doctor signs onto a computerized medical record, the first screen is often a list of alerts. This can be a very long list, and it can include critical information that needs immediate action, such as critical lab results. But this important information is usually buried in a list of irrelevant, unnecessary notices. Many computerized systems do not distinguish between the two.

Allopathic medicine – mainstream medicine, which uses medications, surgery, etc. The term is used to distinguish the practice from homeopathic medicine.

Board certified – credentials attained by a physician who has passed an examination and demonstrated skills in a medical specialty.

Burnout – feelings of exhaustion, low motivation and energy, and frustration, sometimes with decreased work performance, often impacting private family life.

Crowdsource – solving a problem by enlisting a large number of participants.

Direct Primary Care (medical retainer) - a medical practice model which involves a flat monthly fee, which covers whatever services are needed.

EFT, Emotional Freedom Technique – a therapy technique derived from the ancient Chinese system of acupuncture, using tapping on energy points rather than needles.

Emotional resilience – the ability to adapt to stressful situations with no or little difficulty.

Emotional intelligence – the ability to understand emotions, both one's own and those of other people, and to manage those feelings.

Grandfathered – a provision that exempts a group from a new regulation or law. Before, 1990, board certification was granted for life, and those who were already certified at that time were not required to recertify periodically.

MOC, Maintenance of Certification – physicians who were board certified after about 1990 are granted time-limited credentials and required to retest periodically, in order to maintain certification status.

Placebo – anything that is presented as medical treatment, but contains no active ingredient.

Placebo effect (placebo response) – medical studies often compare one group treated with an active medication, with another group treated with an inactive agent, or placebo. In many studies, some patients taking the placebo see improvement in symptoms.

Prior authorization, pre-authorization – before a prescription is written, many insurance companies require approval; otherwise, they will not pay for the medication or procedure.

INDEX

Do You Have Enough Time With Patients?

TO MY DOCTOR:

✓ I am aware that some physicians are frustrated with the lack of time they have with patients, and with many other obstacles to providing quality patient care. Clearly, something needs to be done.

✓ I would like to see this change. I would like to be part of the solution.

✓ What obstacles affect you? Is there anything citizens can do to intervene? What can the general public do to change this?

✓ If you have any suggestions about how patients can help bring back the doctor-patient relationship, I would like to hear them. We can write letters and blogs, make phone calls, and contact local media. We can put pressure on legislators and health care executives. You may have some ideas about other things we can do.

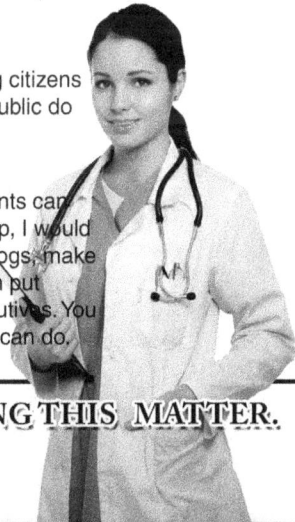

THANK YOU FOR CONSIDERING THIS MATTER.

Let's Fix
HEALTH CARE

For more information, see TheNewOldThing.com

WE CAN CHANGE THIS

TO MY DOCTOR:

☑ The US pays the most for health care of any country in the world, but we are not the healthiest. I believe we can change that.

☑ I understand that when self-healing occurs in medical research, it is dismissed as "placebo response" and the data is ignored. I would like more of our tax money to go toward learning how the body heals itself. I support research into self-healing and the placebo response, and ways to assist healing.

☑ I am in favor of allocating five percent of all biomedical research funding to understanding the placebo effect, both basic and clinical science, and energy medicine.

☑ I believe doctors can make this happen through their local medical society and state legislature. Perhaps you would be willing to help that change.

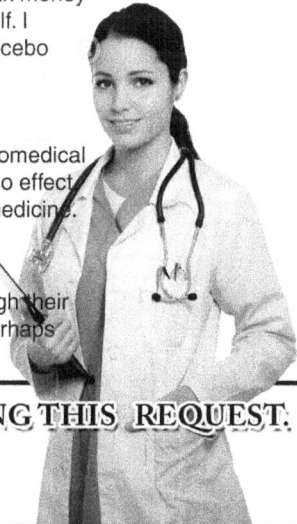

THANK YOU FOR CONSIDERING THIS REQUEST.

Let's ✕ Fix
HEALTH ⚒ CARE

For more information, see TheNewOldThing.com